157
G549M

MENTAL HEALTH OR MENTAL ILLNESS?

MENTAL HEALTH
or
MENTAL ILLNESS?

Psychiatry for Practical Action

by

William Glasser, M.D.

Perennial Library
Harper & Row, Publishers, New York

MENTAL HEALTH OR MENTAL ILLNESS?

INTRODUCTION Copyright © 1970 by William Glasser.

Copyright © 1960 by William Glasser.

Printed in the United States of America.

All rights in this book are reserved. No part of the book may be used or reproduced in any manner whatsoever without written permission except in the case of brief quotations embodied in critical articles and reviews. For information address Harper & Row, Publishers, Incorporated, 49 East 33rd Street, New York, N. Y. 10016.

First PERENNIAL LIBRARY edition published 1970 by
Harper & Row, Publishers, Incorporated,
New York, N. Y. 10016.

*To Mary Perry, Helen Coad,
the Staff, and Girls of Ventura School*

Contents

	PAGE
AUTHOR'S INTRODUCTION	ix
FOREWORD BY MORRIS HERMAN, M.D.	xiii
AUTHOR'S PREFACE	xv

I NORMAL HUMAN FUNCTIONING

Introduction	1
1. The Person and His Needs	3
2. The World, or Reality, or Society	7
3. The Ego—General and Specific Functions—and the Function of Psychiatry	9
4. The Ego Reactions—General and Specific—the Emotions	20
5. Ego Defenses—Unconscious Ego Functions	32
6. Character or Personality—the Pattern of the Ego	39
7. Development of the Ego	42

II ABNORMAL HUMAN FUNCTIONING

Introduction	57
8. Incomplete Ego Functioning—Personality or Character Disorders	59
9. Ego Weakness—Neurotic Ego Functioning—Neuroses	70
10. The Changing Manifestations of Neuroses	76
11. Specific Ego Weakness—Neurotic Symptoms—Symptom Neuroses	79

12.	Generalized Ego Weakness—Anxiety Neuroses	89
13.	Generalized Ego Weakness—Character Neuroses	92
14.	Special Character Neuroses—Sexual Neuroses	100
15.	Ego Thickness, Rigidity, Impenetrability—Psychosis	111
16.	Psychosis—Specific Factors	119
17.	Depression and Psychosomatic Disease	129

III PSYCHIATRIC TREATMENT

	Introduction	141
18.	The People Who Treat	145
19.	The Types of Psychiatric Treatment	149
20.	Problems Inherent in Psychiatric Treatment	155
21.	Psychotherapy	162
22.	Treatments of Patients Who Are in Institutions	169

IV MENTAL HYGIENE

	Introduction	187
23.	Family Mental Hygiene	191
24.	Community Mental Hygiene	199
	Conclusion	204
	INDEX	205

Author's Introduction

This book was written so that any interested person could easily gain a basic understanding of psychology. It was derived from a series of lectures I gave to employees of the California Youth Authority in order to help them work more effectively with the young people they were assigned to rehabilitate. I had in mind also that it would be a helpful book for school teachers, beginning social workers, correctional workers, vocational counselors, nurses, and others whose major effort is with people. This book could also serve as a supplementary text for any high school or beginning college course in psychology.

Part I explains effective behavior or, as I now prefer to call it, responsible or successful behavior. Here, as well as in Part II, where I describe abnormal or, as I now prefer to call it, defective or irresponsible functioning, I use schematic diagrams to explain a variety of familiar behavior. It is important that these diagrams be understood for what they are: aids to understanding. They are not a real part of a person any more than a blueprint is a real part of the building for which it stands.

In Part II I discuss what is loosely, and I believe wrongly, called mental illness. I state in the introduction to Part II that I use these terms only because in 1959 they were so integral a part of our psychological jargon that I thought it would have been confusing to throw them out—a step I did take 5 years later in *Reality Therapy*[1].

---

[1] Glasser, W., *Reality Therapy*, Harper & Row, New York, 1965.

The present reader should appreciate that traditional terms like schizophrenia, neurosis, and character disorder are inaccurate and misleading. They are used here only because unfortunately this is how ineffective, or irresponsible, people are still described in most books or articles in this field.

In Part III, "Psychiatric treatment," is short because the main emphasis of this book is not treatment. In fact, it was this short section which was expanded into the complete book *Reality Therapy*.

Part IV, "Mental hygiene," is more important now than ever. In my suggestions one can see the workings of many self-help organizations, such as Synanon or Recovery, Inc. I do not mean to indicate that these organizations sprang from my thinking; I mean that following this same line of thinking they have prospered and done much good over the last decade. Their success confirms more than ever the need to move in this direction. Toward that goal I have recently devoted myself to working in the public schools for the express purpose of helping more children succeed, and in this success strengthen themselves and improve their ability to cope with their environment. "Schools Without Failure"[2], my most recent book, details this approach, and does so partly through an extension of the basic thinking of Chapter 23 in this book. I am optimistic that this approach will continue to help more people help themselves to a more effective life.

WILLIAM GLASSER, M.D.

May, 1969

---

[2] Glasser, W., *Schools Without Failure*, Harper & Row, New York 1969.

Acknowledgment

I wish to acknowledge and thank the following three persons who contributed so much to this book: G. L. Harrington, M.D., for giving me so much of his valuable time and for his teaching and constant encouragement; Robert L. Glasser for the hundreds of hours spent in editing; Hal Tritel for the illustrations which express the ideas so well.

Foreword

The field of mental health may be considered one of the largest public health areas today. It is well known that one-half the hospital beds in the country are occupied by psychiatric patients. Significant parts of the national, state, and municipal budgets are designated for mental illness and attest to the economic importance of this problem. With the increase in interest and activity in the field of mental health, it has become necessary to define, describe, and elucidate points of view relating to the factors operative in mental health and mental illness.

It is not easy to depict in clear terms the complex and controversial aspects of psychiatry. Everyone who teaches in the field of psychiatry soon becomes aware of the difficulty of expressing cogently the many concepts basic to the understanding of mental processes. It is a great pleasure, therefore, to come upon this book, which so lucidly expounds its ideas.

In order to provide understanding of abnormal mental functioning, it is necessary to give a broad perspective of the human mind and the way in which the human organism is patterned. Dr. Glasser has formulated this by dividing the patterns of the mind into three main categories: the person and his needs, the reality or world, and the ego (the mediator between the person and the world). Essentially the author emphasizes the reactions of the ego—its problems, its vicissitudes, its weakness, its strength. An expertly written section, together with helpful diagrams, makes clear what the author means by the different varieties of ego disturbances.

Perhaps the greatest contribution of this volume is its emphasis on the bold principle that people with only moderately effective ego function can be improved without psychotherapy but by direct and indirect education. A very serious suggestion is made that there be created in the community a mental hygiene agency, not for the treatment of the mentally ill but for the development of more effective egos in families, with special emphasis on the contribution of parents. A community mental hygiene agency would be developed along the educational lines and utilized for governmental groups, clubs, unions, police and welfare departments, and other community organizations. It is stressed that these community mental health agencies are not for treatment but for prevention of illness and improvement of function.

The author has produced a systematic work in the exposition of mental functioning both normal and abnormal. Although he has described patterns of development and factors leading to weak ego formation, it is clear that much research is still needed to answer some of the pertinent questions raised. This book is of aid in pointing out the areas that require further elucidation. It will be particularly useful for workers in the fields of correction, education, and mental health and valuable also for nurses and medical students. It can be read with profit by any intelligent person interested in obtaining information about an important segment of human behavior.

Morris Herman, M.D.
Professor of Psychiatry
New York School of Medicine
New York University Medical Center

Author's Preface

During the past few years I have been lecturing on psychiatry to audiences composed mainly of people who work in institutions within the California Youth Authority. The purpose of the lectures has been to make the concepts of psychiatry understandable to these people so that they might apply the ideas presented to their jobs of working with delinquent adolescents. Initial audiences were skeptical; they seemed to think that the ideas of psychiatry were fine for psychiatrists but of no real use in everyday work with the kids. It was the old story of the theoretical man versus the practical man. In order to break through this resistance I have developed a new conceptual approach to teaching psychiatry which can be easily understood without any previous knowledge of the subject. The response to these lectures delivered to audiences comprised of people with varying degrees of training was extremely gratifying. The psychologically sophisticated people told me that they appreciated the simplicity and clarity of this new conceptual approach, and, more important, the untrained personnel were able to grasp effectively the principles of psychiatry when they were presented in this way.

People to whom I spoke asked me what they could read further to follow up the lectures. In response to these requests I decided that my lecture material would be most meaningful if it were written down, a task which has now culminated in this book.

I feel strongly that the problem of mental illness and abnormal functioning cannot be solved unless more people, having learned about the problem, will take an active part instead of leaving the whole situation in the hands of psychiatrists. There will never be enough psychiatrists to cope with even a small portion of the immense task. It is my hope that this book will help provide information leading to a greater public awareness of the problem of mental illness.

WILLIAM GLASSER, M.D.
Los Angeles, California

I

NORMAL HUMAN FUNCTIONING

Introduction

Exactly what it is that constitutes normal human functioning has been a controversial subject throughout history, probably even more difficult to define than the wide variations of abnormal behavior. The necessary preoccupation with the problems created by abnormal behavior has been stressed to the point where an artificial gap often exists between aberrant and normal functioning. This artificial gap has in turn led to the impression that abnormal is in some way very much different from normal, with the result that in most psychiatric discussions these two concepts are not directly related. Such a dichotomy is unfortunate because the two should not be artificially separated, nor should the concept of what constitutes normal functioning be minimized. *A normal human being is one who functions effectively, has some degree of happiness, and achieves something worthwhile to himself within the rules of the society in which he lives.* To understand in detail how a person successfully achieves this desirable goal, we must start with three distinct, but related criteria:

1. The person and his needs.
2. The world, or the reality, or the society in which the individual lives.
3. The ego—the mediator between the person and the world.

The explanation of these three basic criteria, both individually and as they relate to each other as well as how they can be affected by psychological intervention, is the essential text of this book.

1

The Person and His Needs

EACH PERSON IS BORN WITH A DEFINITE SET OF BASIC NEEDS. From them all the countless variations of individual needs arise. For example, a person may have a strong basic need for love and affection. From this he may develop a need for closeness to many people in order to get love. He may develop a need to enter a certain occupation, such as medicine, where he can be in intimate contact with many people. He may then specialize in pediatrics because with children it seems easier to give and receive love. Later he may go into child psychiatry to work with emotional rather than physiologic problems in order to get more intimate. Each choice along the way is felt as a strong need, each is interrelated, but all arise from the basic need for love. If they are fulfilled, a feeling of satisfaction, release from tension, and ultimately happiness, results. If these strong needs are not satisfied, the person will suffer.

Basic needs do not change with age. Contrary to many beliefs, the basic needs of a newborn infant are the same as those of a twenty-year-old, a fifty- or ninety-year-old. *The needs of all people, normal or abnormal, are the same.* The most maladjusted child has the same needs as a retired minister. *Contact with reality does not change needs.* The most withdrawn psychotic in a mental ward has needs no different from the psychiatrist assigned the task of helping him. *Differences in sex, color, religion, or race do not change needs.* It is quite possible that even higher mammals have roughly the same basic needs as humans. Needs therefore are the same for everyone. What is different is the countless variations by which people satisfy or try to satisfy these needs. For example, to satisfy the need for love, one person may become a psychiatrist, another a philanthropist, a third an alcoholic, and a fourth a "Don Juan." Each in his own way is trying, successfully or unsuccessfully, to satisfy this strong and pressing need.

Basic Needs

There are *two basic groups of needs* which each individual must satisfy. These are:

1. Physiologic needs—food, air, water, warmth, (sex).
2. Psychologic needs—love, social needs, achievement.

Physiologic Needs

Physiologic needs are self-evident. Few people reading this book suffer from a lack of satisfaction of basic physiologic needs: food, water, air, and a proper temperature range. We take the satisfaction of these needs for granted, unless during a period of hardship one or more is remarkably unsatisfied. When one of them goes unfulfilled for any length of time the suffering person becomes filled with fear, struggling desperately, even unreasonably, to satisfy the need. If one of these basic requirements continues to be unsatisfied, the person dies. Although a lack of sexual relations never causes death, this need must be classified as partly physiological. In human beings, however, sexual relationship without love can produce only brief satisfaction. Because it is so intimately related to the psychological needs, it is considered as a part of the need for love.

Psychological Needs

Psychological needs, more complicated than physiological needs, are of equal importance. Although they do not have the extreme urgency of the physiologic needs, they are constantly exerting pressure on every person.

Love and Affection

This need covers the entire range of love and affection from simple, casual friendship to deepest sexual love. We need love and affection throughout our lives. No one is immune to the need to feel that someone cares for him and that he cares for someone else. We become acutely or chronically uncomfortable when we lose the ability satisfactorily to fulfill this need. That infants may die if this need is not satisfied was shown during World War II in Nazi-occupied France. There in large state nurseries babies from one to six months of age began to die mysteriously. Despite the fact that all their physiologic needs were filled, they became listless, would not eat, became stuporous, and died. It was discovered that only those babies who were not anyone's favorite were becoming sick while those favored ones who received a few minutes of loving handling each day thrived. By giving each infant a few minutes of fondling several times a day, the problem almost completely disappeared. Although not conclusive proof, this occurrence is a strong indication that the need for love and affection is so basic that its lack at an early age, when we are dependent on others, can be fatal. We may not die from its lack later on, but we can never be happy when this need is not fulfilled in its complete range from simple affection to sexual love.

Social Needs

Although they are closely related, social needs should be differentiated from the need for love and affection. Almost all people have a need for other people. Sometimes we yearn to "get away from it all," but when we do, we often become lonely. It is an unusual person who can comfortably tolerate any extended period without companionship. Of all the punishments which have endured through the ages, solitary confinement still stands as a cruel testament to this need. Many people who have been isolated voluntarily for long periods of time have reported they hallucinate people who are often friendly and helpful to them.

Admiral Byrd, when he spent the winter alone in Little America, chronicled his hallucinations of other people. Recognizing these visions as a protective measure within his ego to relieve his acute loneliness, he understood that they were not symptoms of insanity. In his travels around the world alone Captain Joshua Slocum had a similar experience in which he described an imaginary companion who steered his boat when he was too ill to hold the tiller. Even though it may come as a painful realization to those who cherish feelings of independence, the fact remains, whether we like it or not, that we need each other.

Achievement

There are many indications that humans have a strong need to achieve something, to have the feeling that they are accomplishing something worthwhile. Even if no praise or love accompanies our achievement, we still strive continually in many directions. Why does a small baby struggle to crawl, to walk, or to explore, a small child strive to read, or an old man whittle or garden? Why does a vigorous older person often wither and become sick when his retirement is enforced from a position of achievement? Why are people altruistically interested in helping others, why do they suffer privation in order to write, paint, or compose? Although the derivatives of this need can become extremely complex, it may be stated that we all have an innate need to feel that we are doing something worthwhile. We have this above and beyond whom we are doing it for and what material reward we may receive. Related to this need is the phenomenon of human curiosity, the desire to explore, to understand the mysteries of the world. Unless in some degree we can satisfy the need for achievement, we suffer. It is unfortunate that individual achievement in our society is in many cases stifled by the structured, organizational environment so well described by W. H. Whyte in his book *The Organization Man*.[1]

[1] W. H. Whyte, Jr., *The Organization Man* (New York: Simon and Schuster, Inc., 1956).

2

The World, or Reality, or Society

THE SECOND OF THE THREE CRITERIA FOR THE UNDERSTANDing of human behavior is the concept of the world around us. The world includes the people and the things which surround all of us. It is in the world that all people must satisfy the two groups of needs previously discussed. How they do this varies, but everyone except a small group of completely psychotic people do it in some way and to some degree.

Initially, what is important to each person is that relatively small segment of the world which surrounds him. He must understand and abide by the rules of this world and learn how his needs can be satisfied in it. If he cannot do this he is in trouble.

It is important to realize that even in the same geographical area the "world" is quite variable. Social rules differ and what is considered correct behavior in one section of a city might horrify a person who lives in another part. In theory each person must obey the same legal rules, but when a person breaks the law the punishment may vary widely. In the South this is graphically exemplified in the case of a Negro and white person breaking the same law, e.g., rape of a person of opposite race. We must therefore understand that the world or reality or society is constant in a very broad sense only. In any particular instance, it may be extremely variable; and it is this variation which is so confusing to the person trying to satisfy his needs. Thus we can see the immediate problem facing the human being in trying to establish a normal pattern. He has constant needs to satisfy. He is given to understand by the many institutions which comprise his environment that the segment of reality which surrounds him is constant, but this is not so. He must always be alert to cope with many variations in the world.

We must examine each person's narrow world—his family and his immediate surroundings which are of prime importance in setting the pattern for the transition to the (common) world. It is through these media that he gains his first knowledge of reality. The more consistent, realistic, and loving the family, the better prepared are the children to face the reality of the unprotected (common) world. Unfortunately, because most families present inconsistent reality patterns to the growing child, the individual has a poor preparation for his graduation to the larger common world.

Thus the world, both in a narrow family sense and in a larger (common) sense, is variable and inconsistent, but it consistently exists this way.

Only a very few remarkable people ever succeed in changing the reality situation. Most of us must either accept existing conditions around us or run from one part of the world to another in an unsuccessful effort to change the world. All that is accomplished is changing physical location or social position. We have not changed reality; we have only changed our position relative to it, and must still fulfill the same needs in our new position. How well we succeed usually determines our willingness to stay in this position. Though our strivings to change the world are illogical, very few of us ever give up trying. We constantly gripe, complain, and struggle with reality, living in hope and fantasy that we, or some miracle, will change our surroundings so that we can better satisfy our needs. Only a few very fortunate people learn from experience that they, not the world, must do the changing. It is the variability and inconsistency of our world which tricks us into thinking that perhaps we can change it. We are often given the illusion that we can change our surroundings when in fact either they change in their own inconsistent pattern and/or we change our position relative to the world.

We continually struggle in the world, goaded by the pressure of our constant needs. That many of us succeed fairly well is testimony to the strength and resiliency of the human ego. Vast numbers, however, do not succeed in this struggle; they can neither satisfy needs in their existing world, nor change the world, nor satisfactorily change their positions in the world. Their failure causes them to become a responsibility for all of us, and our success as a society in some measure depends on how well we discharge this responsibility.

3
❖

The Ego—General and Specific Functions— and the Function of Psychiatry

THE EGO CAN BE BEST DESCRIBED AS THE TOTAL MENTAL functioning of the person. Included are intellectual functioning, emotional functioning, and each individual's unique pattern of reacting called his "personality" or character. The study of what the ego is and does has been the prime subject of psychology and philosophy for ages. Ancient medicine was initially vitally concerned with ego function, but medicine today is more concerned with bodily function, lagging behind in its attempts to understand and relate ego functioning to bodily functioning. The average medical doctor spends little time working out this complex relationship in his patients, most of whom paradoxically come to him with some breakdown in ego functioning. In our society, psychiatrists, psychologists, and social workers are the people who have taken on the task of improving the ego function and preventing ego breakdown. What psychiatry knows and does about poor ego functioning is a mystery to most people, with the result that society either blindly trusts or mistrusts this field. It is therefore incumbent upon psychiatrists not only to work hard at their basic job of developing knowledge about ego functioning but also to dispense this knowledge to the public in a way in which it can be understood.

Although ego functioning is complex, there is a simple way to approach it. The primary functions of the ego are to direct the person so that he may fulfill his needs in the world and protect him as much as possible from any dangers present in the world.

The relationship of the ego to the person and the world can be shown graphically by the following Diagram A.

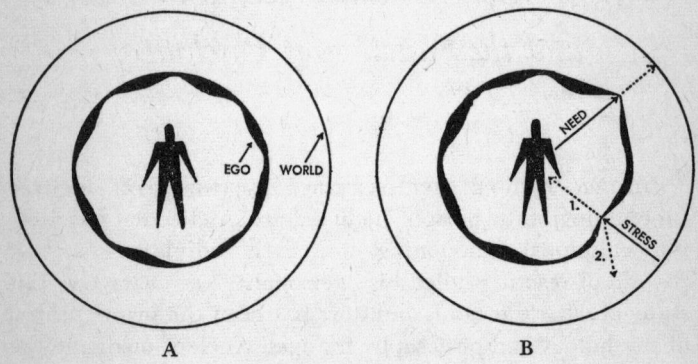

Here we see a small circle which represents a human being with his needs. Outside that is a large circle showing the world or reality surrounding this person. Between these, surrounding the small circle, is a wavy line representing the flexible ego. The ego encircles the person completely, mediating all contacts between him and the world. It both directs him in his quests to fulfill his needs in the world and helps protect the person from any dangers in the world which might harm him. This mechanism may be clarified by reference to the more detailed Diagram B. The outgoing arrows represent needs of the person being mediated by the ego before going into the world. The ingoing arrows represent stresses of the world being mediated before they get to the person. For example: A person has a need to eat. This need is felt by the ego and the ego directs the person to a situation in which food can be obtained. An example of stress is a thirsty person suffering the stress of being lost in a desert without water. If the ego cannot direct the person to an oasis, the stress (Arrow 1) will kill the person, but if he does find an oasis, the ego will successfully cope with the stress (Arrow 2).

For explanatory purposes the example illustrated by Diagram B was extreme; the ego is rarely faced with such rigorous conditions. It immediately and completely fulfills only a few needs, often delays or alters the satisfaction of most needs with the result that some degree of partial fulfillment generally occurs. A teen-age boy who saved his money to attend a burlesque show illustrates the ego's task of delaying, altering, and partially fulfilling the need for sex. The same variation works for stresses; some it completely wards off, others are delayed, but many, even though delayed, are only partially warded off. The degree of urgency, increased stress, painful preparation, and waiting for a grade, all occurring between the time a term paper is assigned and completed, illustrates this process. Depending on its basic strength, the ego, twenty-four hours a day, awake and asleep, fulfills the needs and protects the person as successfully as possible. To do this job the human ego has developed into a complex psychological system which man for ages has struggled to understand. The task, however, when reduced to its basic dimensions is very simple—*fulfill the needs and keep the person alive.* How well any ego succeeds is a measure of that person's psychological success, or a measure of how effectively his ego functions. At this time let us redefine a "normal" person as one whose ego functions well enough to satisfy reasonably his basic and derived needs—which in turn produces that good feeling called happiness—and to protect him from dangers.

Using a parallel definition, we say that an abnormal person has an ego which does not do this job successfully. This failure is reflected by varying amounts of abnormal behavior or suffering, or both. It is the function of psychiatrists in our society to aid abnormal ego functioning to become more normal. At this point, the use of the term "normal" will be discontinued because normal carries with it a statistical connotation meaning average with the implied meaning of similarity. *Normal will be replaced with the word effective and abnormal with defective.* People with a normal or *effective ego* may be almost totally dissimilar even as people with an abnormal or *defective ego* may be dissimilar. An Australian bushman and an English peer may both have good, strong, effective ego functioning within the world in which they live, yet no two people could be less alike. It must be remembered that effective ego functioning need not mean similar functioning. The person with an effective ego has the ability to conform, but is not compelled to comply with any standard of conformity beyond that which he may choose for himself. It would be wrong to construe the task of psychiatry to be the molding of any patient into a hypothetical "normal" person. The goal of the psychiatrist is only to help the patient establish more effective ego functioning in those areas where his ego function is defective.

Finally a word about the relationship of the world to the effective ego. Theoretically the person with an effective ego would fulfill his needs and protect himself under all conditions of the world or reality. Actually, such cases are rare. Few of us could survive under conditions which the Australian aborigine might consider optimum, and most of us suffer if we are forced to make any great changes in our world such as conscription into the military. In time and with some luck people with an effective ego adjust to new conditions. There are, however, vast numbers who, never having this test, function effectively in their small segment of a relatively constant reality from birth to death. How strong these egos are is a hypothetical question, often argued by psychologists, but not relevant to the main problem which exists today. We are primarily concerned with people whose ego is defective under conditions which are not excessively stressful. As psychiatrists we rarely treat a patient whose problem stems from a bad reality situation. The majority of patients suffer from defective egos, unable to cope well with any reality situation, good, bad, or indifferent. Therefore, we might amend the function of psychiatry to that of making defective ego functioning into effective ego functioning within a reasonably tolerable reality situation.

Specific Ego Functions

In addition to the over-all general functions of the ego, which are to protect the person and fill his needs, there are three primary specific ego functions. These are:

1. Identity—establishing in ego the feeling of I AM I.
2. Judgment—testing reality.
3. Aggressiveness—forceful ego activity.

Identity

The most important ego function is that of establishing identity. This means the integration into the ego of a clear, strong, positive feeling of I AM I. All human behavior, reactions, emotions, striving, are directed, in a basic sense, toward the furthering of the feeling of personal identity. If we know who we are, we think very little about this ego function. We know who we are in relation to that segment of the world in which we live. We identify ourselves with reference to familiar people and surroundings. If placed in a different situation where all is unfamiliar, we try first of all to establish who we are. If we are unable to do this, we become frightened, anxious, and often immobilized. When we cannot establish our identity, we suffer what is probably the most upsetting of all human experiences. We do not establish this ego function easily, in many cases struggling all our lives to establish who we are in the world.

An effective ego is one in which there is a strong sense of identity. The feeling of I AM I is built into the ego with enough strength to remain unshaken by changes in the world. An effective ego is one which can efficiently fulfill needs because it knows for whom it is performing this task. It is satisfying the needs of a *definite, identified* person. The relationship is analogous to building a house from a detailed set of plans or specifications. Each step could be carefully planned because the final result, the identity of the finished product, is clearly established. Defective egos function inefficiently because there is only a poorly defined sense of identity. It is hard to satisfy the needs when there is only a poor concept of whose needs these are. This may be likened to building a house from a few rough sketches, or from vague ideas in the head of the future occupant. Inefficient, wasteful, repetitious labor is a necessary accompaniment to such a project.

First and foremost an effective ego establishes sexual identity. For effective functioning a person must know clearly what his sex is. This statement in no way implies that the popular Hollywood version of masculine–feminine is an example of a successful identification. It means that whatever the outward characteristics may be, the person with an effective ego knows what his sex is. A gentle, sensitive, considerate man may have a more solid sense of maleness than a pugnacious, aggressive, bemuscled, athletic type, considered so masculine in our sexually confused society. Successful identification includes the establishment of correct body identity or body image. This image exists in the ego, that is, the person has a clear, definite picture of his body and accepts what he sees. He feels that his body is masculine, or in the case of a woman, feminine. Realizing that the sexual organs are functional, he or she derives great satisfaction from normal sexual love, feeling neither danger nor inferiority because of sexual functions. The more definite the picture of his or her physical sexual image and its functions, the more effective is the ego in establishing identity.

An effective ego is one that has a well-established set of values or ideals in which the person strongly believes. These values are attained in many situations where choices must be made. In the establishing of strong positive identity these choices are made. For example: A person may consider himself honest beyond question until a definite test of his honesty occurs. He may find a wallet, with no identification, containing a large sum of money. He now has the choice of attempting to find the owner to return the money or saying nothing. At this time, when he makes his choice, his values are established, and his identity solidified with respect to honesty.

Much of what many people conceive to be good in our world has been wrought by individuals who were willing under pain and pressure to stand for what they thought was right—their personal values. They were not willing to change their beliefs for a different, more comfortable identity. They knew who they were and were not afraid to state their beliefs. People who know who they are rarely straddle the fence, but if they do, at least they know they are astride.

A good sense of identity implies knowing where you are in respect to time, place, and social environment. A person with a good sense of identity knows the dimensions of his world and where he stands relative to them.

These are all components of the function of identity established at great effort for the individual, but only when this ego function is established can needs be efficiently satisfied. In the discussion of defective ego functioning the lack of a sense of identity will be related to many psychiatric problems present in our society.

JUDGMENT

In order to have effective ego functioning it is necessary that the ego be able to test efficiently the world of reality so that it may find those areas of the world which may best satisfy the needs of the person, and to recognize those areas which might harm him. Testing reality, which includes the function of judgment, means an ability to understand the rules of the world and society. Thus, the ego must fulfill its needs yet stay within the rules of the world. In juvenile delinquents, the ego, functioning to fulfill needs, does so in a way which breaks the laws or rules. This procedure is inefficient because the punishment which follows serves to frustrate other needs, often in excess of any satisfaction gained. Neurotic people who may have faulty ability to test reality, characteristically are afraid to fulfill needs because their egos misperceive a portion of the world as dangerous when it is not, e.g., a man who exhausts himself climbing stairs because he is frightened of elevators.

It takes energy to exercise judgment and make decisions. Many people prefer to have others do this for them because of the mental labor involved as well as the fact that the end result, even of good judgment, may be painful at times. Effective ego functioning embodies the ability to exercise good judgment, to test reality even at the expense of physical or mental pain. Examples of this would be returning from a wonderful vacation when strong forces say, "Stay," or enduring the pain of dental work rather than postponing it and perhaps losing a tooth.

A very important part of testing reality is the concept of time. We need to accept and adjust to the fact that the world runs on schedule. Only a few rich and/or eccentric people or primitive people can dispense with the idea of time and the clock. As an aborigine said to the anthropologist, "We have no god which we obey to the point that you follow the god strapped to your wrist." Whether we like it or not, time is a dimension of our reality which our egos must appreciate. We must also understand that there is a certain order in the world which most people accept that has to do with the passage of time. For example, we may be in love when we are sixteen, but it will be better to wait until we are older to get married. Although we may have to delay the immediate fulfilling of needs, we can, with planning and judgment, satisfy them later. We must be able to delay satisfactions, using our ego to place our needs in the proper perspective with regard to time. People who do not understand this concept do well only as long as others are tolerant of their lack. For example, no one expects a small child to wait patiently until his next birthday for a certain desired object. If he is forced to wait, he suffers because he has no concept of the time involved, whereas a sixteen-year-old may wait, albeit impatiently, until he becomes eighteen for a car because he is able to understand the time differential. If the teen-ager has poor ego functioning with respect to time he may steal a car, blaming his parents, who he feels made him wait longer than he could tolerate. He is then in serious trouble, partly because his ego functioning was defective in this respect, although other factors are usually involved. There are endless examples, the latter being a most familiar one. The important concept here is that as we mature we must have an accurate working sense of time. If this ego function is defective serious trouble may ensue.

Aggressive Behavior

The final basic specific ego function is that of forceful aggressive behavior. It is common to all animals, man certainly included, to behave forcefully in the satisfaction of needs. An effective ego is necessarily forceful and aggressive, in contrast to passivity or apathy, which may be exhibited when this ego function is defective.

Most of the rules of our world have been devised in order to regulate the extremes of this ego function. In our modern "civilized" world we are expected to limit our aggressiveness to the point where others are not harmed. All civilized societies are continually caught in a basic dilemma: the need to curb aggressiveness to the point where it does not harm others yet not curb it to the point where it ceases to function for the good of the individual. Societies in which this ego function has been lost soon fall prey to other societies where aggression is a usual and accepted mode of behavior. The invasion and conquest of the peaceful Chinese by Genghis Khan is typical of many historical examples of this occurrence.

In our society (up until recently) individual aggression was considered to be a masculine function. Females, as they reached puberty, supposedly relinquished this ego function to the male as it was his prerogative to exhibit such behavior. In reality, however, this was only a superficial relinquishment because the female expected the man to be aggressive not only for himself but for his woman. The males acted as the instrument of the female aggressive ego function; this was the accepted way. When population was sparser, it was easier for males to do this. Vast increases in population, with the subsequent increase in rules and regulations, made it more difficult for the male to be the aggressive instrument for himself and for his woman. Medical advances have prolonged female lives to the point where women outnumber males; thus there is no man to be aggressive for increasing numbers of women. Therefore, with these changes, the pattern has changed so that now women directly express aggressive behavior, to the consternation of many who do not accept this fact easily. Although we may wish to recall the good old days when woman was superficially passive, we must recognize that those days are gone forever. Woman will continue to express this ego function unless she has a man strong enough to do it for her.

This type of man, while still present in great numbers, is on the wane. Male aggressiveness is declining for at least two reasons: (1) the rules are too strict now; it's hard enough to be aggressive for yourself, let alone for your woman; and (2) the men have found out it is easier for them to let the woman fight her own battles. Some women have even reversed the role, as in some of our TV family series where the woman becomes the instrument for her own aggressiveness as well as her man's.

The sooner the psychological professions accept the basic fact that aggression is a common ego function capable of being expressed by man for woman, woman for man, or each for himself, the sooner much of the present turmoil concerning sexual aggressiveness will be dissipated.

As the method in which aggression is expressed changes from the classical male role, much tension and trouble accrues. Many people, both men and women, are seeking psychiatric care because of an inability properly to express this basic ego function. Those who try to change things back to the way they were are doomed to failure. Psychiatrists need to be the first to recognize that times have changed and that each individual, man or woman, must exercise this ego function in the world in which he lives in an acceptable way.

4

The Ego Reactions—General and Specific— the Emotions

General—The Emotions

THE EGO, IN PERFORMING ITS GENERAL AND SPECIFIC FUNCtions, develops a variety of reactions which can all be classed under the heading of emotions. Thus *emotions are not a basic ego function, but rather the feeling which accompanies the performance of basic ego functions*.

Although emotions are primarily psychological, in all cases they diffuse into physical feelings. Good emotions are accompanied by a sense of physical well-being, muscular relaxation, or pleasant degrees of tension. We feel warm, strong, and physically confident in our body and its ability to function. In contrast the unpleasant emotions are accompanied by a variety of uncomfortable physical reactions. We feel our muscles become tense, our mouth becomes dry, our hands perspire; gastrointestinal upset is common and headache and backache occur frequently. Our bodies feel generally weak which leads to lack of confidence in our physical functioning.

Emotions are extremely important because, under conditions of effective ego functioning, they serve as the reward for this function. Thus we experience pleasant feelings, a variety of good emotions when our ego is effective. Even further, the memory of pleasant feelings or the anticipation of even more intense pleasure can serve as an incentive toward more effective ego functioning in the future.

The answer to the basic question of why the ego continuously struggles to fill the person's never-ending needs is now complete. Previously it was stated that it did so because unsatisfied needs produced a state of displeasure or tension, but this is at best a negative incentive. If displeasure were the only incentive then much human behavior would be inexplicable. It would explain only obvious need-filling activity, but human beings in our culture have progressed far beyond the basic needs. Cultural progress has been made because man is able to receive a positive psychological reward in his ability to experience the variety of rich and satisfying emotions which accompany complex, effective ego functioning. All that is mature, artistic, creative, philosophical, intellectual arises from the achievement or the anticipation of a variety of positive emotions.

When a person has defective ego functioning, he is necessarily limited in his emotional reactions. He has no background of rich emotional experience to serve as an incentive for better ego functioning. He may experience primarily unpleasant feelings to the point where, in many cases, he learns to limit his ego functioning severely in order to avoid the concomitant discomfort. Such a person is flat and unemotional because he functions poorly; life is not easy or pleasant for him. In his attempt to remedy this situation his ego tries many different courses that produce a variety of unpleasant, even haphazard, emotional reactions. Called emotional disturbance, the behavior and feeling which we observe in this type of person is almost always evidence of a serious defect in ego functioning.

Thus, as in its functions, the ego can exhibit a wide pattern of emotional reactions varying from effective, mature, positive reactions to defective, immature, primitive reactions. It can be seen that the type of emotions a person exhibits can serve as a good yardstick for measuring ego function. This correlation is the basis of almost all the psychological tests which measure personality, such as the Rorschach[1] and T.A.T.[2] In describing a person we almost always find most meaningful a description of his emotions. We react to each other's emotions more than to anything else. We are comfortable in the presence of a warm, emotional person and uncomfortable in the presence of a coldblooded, unemotional person. Usually we can easily distinguish between appropriate control of emotions which is mature, and flatness or lack of emotions which we find unpleasant in others. Often we are attracted to people who are able to experience emotions which we cannot feel. We are striving constantly to experience new and richer emotions as our ego grows and matures into a more effective functioning entity.

No attempt will be made here to categorize all of the various emotions. Although this listing has been done by various psychologists, it serves little real purpose. Anyone can understand that all emotions are derivatives of two basic ego reactions: pleasure and displeasure. By the time of birth these nonspecific ego reactions have been established, and from them all other feelings develop. Although pleasurable emotions are important, they do not require explanation beyond the previously stated fact that they accompany effective ego functioning. There are, however, four specific unpleasant ego reactions which, occurring in all people, are basic to the understanding of how human beings function. These are *anxiety, emptiness, hostility,* and *depression*. Although these ego reactions are most important in the understanding of psychiatric disturbance, they are often misunderstood as being the *source* of the disturbance. They are never the source, but rather the

---

[1] Rorschach, a psychological test to assess personality in which the subject's reactions to standard inkblots are evaluated by the psychologist in order to determine the kind of personality the subject has.

[2] Thematic Apperception or T.A.T., a test similar to the Rorschach except standard pictures are used and the subject is asked to make up a story about each picture. From these stories the psychologist determines the subjects' psychological make-up.

ANXIETY

Anxiety is the most general of the ego reactions, occurring in all people, because the ego is never able to satisfy all its general need-filling and protective functions. Everyone experiences anxiety of various intensity for various periods from birth to death. Anxiety may be described as fear, discomfort, uneasiness, guilt, apprehension, or remorse. (These terms are all used under anxiety because their separation is usually artificial, confusing rather than clarifying its meaning). Produced by real or unreal situations, anxiety, if severe in either case, is usually accompanied by a variety of uncomfortable physical feelings typified by muscular tension, gastrointestinal distress, headache, and excessive perspiring. Anxiety produced by a real situation is the painful discomfort and fear of starving of a man lost in the wilderness, whereas anxiety produced by an unreal situation is the intense fright some people experience when they ride in an elevator. We even differentiate between the real and unreal situation by calling the former a fear and the latter a phobia. In the former case the most effective ego may not be able to get a man out of a bad situation, although his ability to survive will be largely measured by how effectively his ego functions in this dangerous reality situation. In the case of the man in the elevator there is no real danger, but his ego mistakenly perceives the situation as dangerous with resultant anxiety. *Thus, you feel or react to how your ego perceives the reality situation, not to the reality of the situation as others might see it.*

People whose egos are defective are often overwhelmed by anxiety and seek psychiatric care. As the ego is strengthened in the psychiatric relationship the anxiety diminishes to more comfortable levels.

Many people, however, suffer from extremely defective

ego functioning yet experience little or no anxiety. This phenomenon will be explained in detail later in the book, but the general principle involved states *that in order to have anxiety, there must be a minimal degree of ego function.* Juvenile delinquents often express no feeling whatever while exhibiting behavior which would be extremely anxiety producing for most people. An example would be "toughs" who participate in a gang killing who, even when caught, say that they feel little except (the secondary fear) that they might now be punished. This can be explained only on the basis that their ego is so defective that there is not enough ego to feel anxiety. They are unable to understand why others are so disturbed, often asking what all the fuss is about? Although unfortunately this serious situation is not uncommon, our society is poorly prepared to deal with it. Punishment is futile because it is effective only if it can reinforce built-in anxiety or remorse. The only solution is to increase ego function so that such behavior will not occur.

Anxiety, like all ego reactions, has a purpose. Within certain limits anxiety serves notice to the ego that, consciously or unconsciously, it is not functioning properly. People with effective ego functioning are goaded by anxiety toward more effective use of their ego. As a warning, however, anxiety is effective only when the ego can remedy its ways. In certain psychiatric disturbances, mainly neuroses, the person may be overwhelmed by anxiety yet have an ego which is unable either to cope with or tolerate anxiety. What serves as a warning to a person with effective ego function becomes a constant source of misery to a person with less effective function. Thus anxiety, unpleasant as it may be, is not in itself good or bad, but serves a definite purpose. What is important is how our egos function in relation to this purpose.

Emptiness

Emptiness is a specific ego reaction which accompanies the failure of the ego to establish identity. It is felt by a person who has a poorly developed sense of I AM I. People who are empty have accompanying physical symptoms of apathy, fatigue, and a general "washed out" feeling. Emptiness is a self-descriptive term. This rather common ego reaction in our society implies a feeling of nothingness, lack of personal worth or esteem, lack of confidence in oneself as a person. In the concept of David Riesman,[3] it indicates a lack of "inner direction." The individual lacks a feeling of self-worth which is not dependent on others. To depend on others for self-worth, e.g., other-directed people, is a compromise which works for many people only as long as they stay in a social situation where such other people exist.

Emptiness is so exceedingly uncomfortable that people strive in many ways to gain relief. A common way is to become hostile, forcing recognition for this behavior. If the hostility does not break the rules of society, some success will accompany this reaction. If it does break the rules, then the individual may pay the high price of retaliation or punishment. Strangely enough, many people and most juvenile delinquents are willing to pay this price as long as even for short periods they are relieved of the feeling of emptiness.

Emptiness implies a lack of fantasy, or imagination, a poverty of what might be described as rich inner life. To the empty person the world is without rewards, life is dull and humdrum. "Kicks" or satisfactions have no inner or built-in foundations, but rather must occur, if at all, in reacting with either people or something else in the environment. Often this takes the form of reacting against a known retaliating force, as in the case of an individual who breaks the law to force the police to punish him, painful as this usually is. The concept that something, even pain, is better than nothing, is very important in understanding how empty people, typified by juvenile delinquents, struggle to avoid this feeling.

[3] David Riesman, *The Lonely Crowd* (New Haven: Yale University Press, 1950).

Angry and unable to entertain themselves, people who are empty often exhibit erratic, unpredictable behavior when this feeling gets too strong. They can't seem to get from life that which they want; they are the gripers, the continual seekers, the people searching for the magic key.

People afflicted with emptiness as a result of poor identity often seek out other identities where they can be more fulfilled. They may compensate by playing the big man when they feel nothing inside. The bully and the self-appointed big shot are examples. "Beatniks" are a current example of a group who are searching for their identity. Others in this quest may vary from role to role; actors are classic examples of people using their profession to gain satisfaction not as themselves, but as different characters whom they can play successfully. The school of method acting teaches the actor to lose himself in his role, to *be* the other person. Using this method may be pathological for actors with a poor sense of identity. James Dean was a good although tragic example of the actor's use of his role; paradoxically he served as a model for many who were searching to find their own identity. To escape from their own deep feelings of emptiness many tried desperately to identify with Dean. When he died, his followers, assaulted by new feelings of emptiness which left them temporarily in limbo, tried to escape by refusing to acknowledge his death.

Almost all people who seek psychiatric help do so partly because of emptiness. They look to the psychiatrist to supply in a measure what they lack, and in proper psychiatric treatment he does this. When the patient finally begins to establish a real feeling of identity, the empty feeling leaves and the person begins to become alive and vital. He begins to function more effectively, establishing new ego patterns which lead to new relationships. As this process occurs, the psychiatrist is gradually released, becoming less important as new relationships take over.

Thus, two important specific ego reactions are anxiety

and emptiness, both important yardsticks of ego functioning. The patient, as he achieves more effective ego function, complains less and less about them. One difference is that the more defective the ego, the more extreme the feeling of emptiness, whereas anxiety, severe as it is, requires a minimal degree of ego function. There is no more certain indication of grossly defective ego functioning than the feeling of emptiness, the lack of all sense of I AM I.

Hostility and Anger—Destructive Feelings

Third in the specific ego reactions are the emotions anger and hostility. These reflect poor ego function and are a usual accompaniment to feelings of frustration when the ego is unable to perform its proper functions.

Why are juvenile delinquents so angry? What are they protesting? These questions are asked because there seems to be no logic in the extremes of anger displayed in gang beatings, lootings, and property destruction. These delinquents exhibit insensitivity to suffering, both their own and that which they cause others. The child or adult involved has poor control or none at all over the emotion—intense anger—that dominates him.

The question can now be partially answered. The anger arises as a reaction to poor ego functioning. People who have effective ego functioning rarely, if ever, display wanton, aggressive feelings. They don't because they are automatically rewarded with satisfying or positive ego reactions which are rich and varied. This is not to say that people with effective egos do not feel anger or hostility, but rather that after a reasonable time they are able to (1) control themselves until it passes; (2) express the anger in a socially acceptable way; or (3) overcome the frustration which caused the anger.

Uncontrolled anger is extremely upsetting in our society. We have built both walls and rules for the express purpose of controlling anger, but the more walls we build, the more we avoid facing the basic problem. Erecting jails, detention homes, and institutions is a negative solution. Monuments to our inability to develop methods of making defective egos more effective, they at best temporarily control socially inacceptable anger. This control, a necessary first step, can never by itself solve the problem. We must accept the fact that anger is here to stay; we can't legislate against it. The only solution is to control it internally, within the angry person. External controls can never solve the problem.

In contrast to the other specific ego reactions, anxiety and emptiness, anger is much less specific, but because of its destructiveness it is socially much more important. It is less specific because it can occur as a reaction to a reaction. For example, the feeling of emptiness, an ego reaction itself, often leads to angry, destructive behavior. The feeling of anxiety also may cause angry behavior or expression. These two sequences demonstrate the further important principle that the emotions usually react among themselves. Emotions breed emotions; an intense ego reaction of any type, pleasurable or unpleasurable, may lead to other reactions. In defective ego functioning this process often occurs with unpleasurable reactions haphazardly generating feelings which the person is not prepared to handle. In more effective ego functioning this interaction also occurs but it happens less with the unpleasant emotions and more in the production of positive, pleasant emotional feelings.

Thus, anger is an ego reaction which occurs not only as a direct consequence of poor ego functioning as do anxiety or emptiness, but also may occur along with any unpleasant feeling. It may lead to actions which cause more unpleasantness, continuing to build up until externally controlled. Eventually antisocial anger is controlled, but not until some members of our society have suffered or died in the interim between the violent expression of the anger and its control. Probably no more gruesome illustration of this process can be cited than the case of Charles Starkweather, recently executed for thirteen senseless murders. Finally, it should be understood that anger is the most difficult reaction to control because, even as it builds up within an individual, it builds up between people. When we control angry people, we often do it with more anger—legal perhaps, but still anger. We react in this way because many of us have not reached the level of effective ego functioning that would allow us to do otherwise. From a social standpoint, a good measure of effective ego functioning is how a society treats angry behavior or even more specifically, how correctional institutions treat angry people consigned to them for custody. We no longer beat and torture people in institutions because we recognize that it does not help them and often endangers us. If it did help, it would still be going on, for even now we hear talk of reinstating corporal punishment in the schools, an open admission that we do not understand the problem. Corporal punishment will work only if the person who is punished has some positive feeling toward the person doing the punishing. For this good feeling to occur the person being punished must have some degree of effective ego functioning. For those who can't control their angry feelings because of defective ego functioning, corporal punishment is useless and even dangerous because it increases the anger. An example of this is Quasimodo in *The Hunchback of Notre Dame*.[4] The basic principle is that anger is an ego reaction with its origin in defective ego functioning. Egos cannot be forced, beaten, or kicked into functioning effectively. We need fewer, not more, external controls if our society is to progress. We must learn more about the ego, how it functions and how defective ego functioning can be corrected. This is the only solution to the problem. Admittedly this solution, which stands on the side of treatment as opposed to punishment and isolation, is difficult.

---

[4] Quasimodo, the hunchback of Notre Dame in the book by Victor Hugo, withdrew in anger and fright after he was senselessly flogged, senseless because he had no ability to understand the reason.

Much of the present "treatment," justified on the grounds of expediency, is directly thwarting this necessary goal.

Depression

Depression is an ego reaction which is not easily described in other words. We say we are depressed or getting depressed or coming out of a depressed state. We are dejected during this state, we are apathetic, we experience a feeling of not caring about anything or anybody. We function poorly, finding it difficult or impossible to work. We lack enthusiasm, *joie de vivre*. Even our actual physical and physiologic functioning is reduced. We are at low ebb, suffering during a state of depression from almost total immobilization of our ego. It neither functions nor reacts except in a very minimal way.

All people experience depression in varying degrees as a usual although unpleasant ego reaction. Most experience it as a transient state, soon recovering from this feeling. In these cases depression is only another ego reaction, but if it continues for a long period of time it is then a mental illness also called depression. The difference between the transient ego reaction which we all feel at times and the mental illness is in severity and duration; the process is the same. This process or mechanism of depression is a very specific type of ego reaction, that is, *depression is a reaction to another strong ego reaction—anger*.

Depression occurs when the ego is unable to express anger either to the outside world or inwardly to the body. The anger then must be contained within the ego itself. The process of the anger being absorbed back into the same ego in which it originated is felt as depression. The strong angry reaction attacks its own source, its own ego, and is experienced in this self-destructive way as depression. In the process the ego is immobilized, and remains so until eventually the anger is dissipated and the depression lifts. Again, if this series of events is short-lived, we have only the emotion or ego reaction called depression or de-ing procedure said that the main thing which kept them from accepting the new identity was conscious repetition of the ideals for which they stood. This part of their identity, ordinarily beneath awareness, was preserved by reliving consciously the factors which went into the establishment of the strong identity.

Thus although much of our ego functioning takes place at a level beneath our *usual* awareness, this ego activity is not unconscious. *Unconscious ego activity takes place at a level beneath our ability to bring it into consciousness.* When people talk about the "unconscious," they are really talking about their preconscious, that mental activity which takes place just beneath awareness. We are never directly aware of our unconscious, although this part of our ego comprises a very important part of our total mental functioning. It is in the unconscious, beneath any awareness that the ego defenses, which comprise the major part of the unconscious part of the ego, function to defend the conscious and preconscious parts of the ego. The ego defenses protect the ego by performing the following tasks:

1. They defend the ego against many pressures and dangers of the world, both major and minor.
2. They defend the ego against excessive pressures generated internally by the constant strong needs.
3. They aid the ego in doing its job efficiently and serve to regulate its functions.

In performing these three jobs the unconscious ego allows the ego to be free from a myriad of irritations and distractions, enabling it to devote its energy toward the conscious fulfillment of its general and specific functions. The ego defenses may be likened to a group of good secretaries and assistants working for a busy executive. They take care of all but the most pressing and urgent business for him. They screen people who might disrupt his work. They are sensitive to his needs, carefully regulating his world so that he can perform his job with great efficiency.

In medicine, the good surgical team contributes the same help to the busy surgeon. Only when they are absent is the surgeon aware of how excellently they do their jobs. He is aware of the fact that they are functioning, but is rarely consciously aware of exactly how they function. In both of these cases, businessman and surgeon, the training of the assistants usually has been done carefully and completely by the man whom they now aid so efficiently. Once he completes their training they function, for him, autonomously. He is now acutely aware of them only when on occasion they fail to function.

The previous examples are analogous to the operation of the ego defenses. Initially most of what is now done automatically and smoothly was done consciously with little of its present efficiency. The ego, in its initial task of directing the child in his efforts to walk, performed with great effort, driven by its need for achievement of which walking was a major challenge early in life. Now each person walks automatically, perhaps only conscious of this activity when in unfortunate circumstances as, for example, when under the influence of alcohol he is asked to prove his sobriety by walking a straight line. Under these conditions he may become painfully aware of how this unconscious ego function, now poisoned by alcohol, has failed to perform up to its usual standard.

The ego defenses gather the memory of extremely painful incidents into the unconscious, leaving us with a memory primarily geared to the conscious recollection of the pleasant aspects of most experiences. Common examples of this are servicemen who, remembering the fun and frolic of their service careers, are hard pressed as years pass to remember the dismal side. The surgeon who in times of disaster operates continually for twenty-four to thirty-six hours until he collapses of exhaustion is protected by powerful defenses from feeling pain or fatigue, or even from suffering loss of skill until a final physical limit is reached. Even in sleep the ego defenses are active by producing dreams, whose major purpose is to protect the needed sleep. We often dream of food, of sexual situations, or the need to urinate when unsatisfied needs in these areas stimulate the ego into the dream activity. To some extent the dream relieves the ego of the task of consciously satisfying these pressures, temporarily replacing the actual need satisfaction and maintaining undisturbed sleep as long as possible. The above are all general examples of the function of the ego defenses, which work day and night to free the ego for important tasks at hand by warding off painful distractions, making complicated physical activities automatic, and reducing intense physiologic pressures which might disturb us.

Specific Ego Defenses

There are two important categories of specific ego defenses. These are the good ego defenses, grouped under the major heading of sublimation, and the poor ego defenses, grouped under denial.

Sublimation

Sublimation is taking an alternate course which partially or completely satisfies a need when one is not able to take a more direct course. This definition implies that not only are basic needs sublimated but also that derivatives of basic needs can be sublimated. Even sublimations can be further sublimated.

Again I refer to the example used earlier in this book when derivatives of needs were cited. In that case, a man who has a direct need for love and affection sublimated part of this by becoming a doctor, then a pediatrician, and finally a child psychiatrist. If he has no awareness of the course which he has taken to get intimacy and love, his ego defenses are operating. They have helped steer his ego into operating consciously to satisfy his need for love, but at the same time, by use of a series of sublimations, he is completely unaware of what his ego defenses have done. If he is aware of what has happened, as he well may be, it is conscious ego functioning and not ego defenses; few people, however, become completely aware of all the factors which determine their occupation. People often become aware of defective ego functioning only through pain, when the ego defenses fail. Thus, if the person in the example has personality characteristics which make him a poor child psychiatrist, the attempt at sublimation will not be satisfactory. He may then seek the aid of another psychiatrist, who will help him become aware of his ego defenses as well as his initial motivation. With help he may be able to improve his conscious ego functioning to the point where he can obtain love more directly, doing away with the need for such extensive sublimation. Because he is now able to fulfill his need outside his occupation he will perform his job more successfully due to strengthened ego functioning, with all the rich emotional rewards therein.

The Roman crowd at the gladiator duels, as well as the American throng at the prize fight or football games, sublimate aggression into socially acceptable channels. The interest that bullfighting has created in modern America is an example of our need for gory channels in which to sublimate our innate aggressiveness in the satisfaction of some needs. We further sublimate by identifying with characters in movies, books, and plays.

In some respects there is a touch of James Thurber's Walter Mitty in all of us; this type of fantasy, however, works only for a limited time. If we depend too much on such sublimations we suffer because at times we must directly fill certain needs; too much sublimation will lead, as it did in the case of Walter Mitty, to unreality which borders on denial. Furthermore, certain needs cannot be sublimated. These are the physiologic needs and the physiologic aspect of the need for sex. We must have food, air, water, and warmth. There are no substitutes for these needs as there is no substitute for normal sexual relations; lack of the latter will not, however, lead to the direct serious consequences of the lack of other physiologic needs. On the positive side, sublimation by the use of a variety of emotionally rewarding alternates and courses help bring out inner capacities which might never appear if all needs were directly satisfied. Woe to the child whose mother fulfills all his needs directly, leaving his ego with nothing except an ability to vegetate. Sublimation is thus a good and important ego defense; the ability to sublimate is part of an effective ego.

Denial

All the poor ego defenses can be grouped under the heading of denial. The person denies that a basic need, or a derivative of a basic need, exists. In this denial he also may deny the existence of the world, an ego function, or an emotion. What he actually does is to deny internal reality, or external reality, or part of his own ego, either singly or in combination. This extremely common defense has three important variations. These are repression, projection, and rationalization, all first cousins of denial.

In small children it is not unusual for the belief that Santa Claus is real to be unshakable. He is real because the child, perhaps to fulfill some need for love, cannot accept any alternative. By repressing the obvious fact that there is no Santa Claus, adults often carry this belief into old age, frequently perpetuating it in their children for probably the same reason that they still believe. We all rationalize that it was not we who did a poor job, but that our failure was caused by a series of unfortunate events beyond our control. We project our failure onto someone else, saying, for example, that the boss is prejudiced against people over forty-five, while at the same time being completely, even vehemently, unaware of our failure to do the job well. These are our ego defenses in action, protecting us against the truth—the truth being that our egos are not capable of effective functioning to fulfill our needs in the situation.

Unfortunately denial is a defense which is almost always

harmful to the welfare of the person. The alcoholic may rationalize his drinking and the gambler his gambling, to the ruin of himself or his family. Whole groups of people suffer, as do the Negroes in the South, partially because of a massive and accepted use of denial. The prejudice and aggression against the Negro is justified by the false rationalization that the Negro is inferior. The massive denial is necessary to keep from awareness a growing fear among the prejudiced that the Negro is just as good as anyone else. This cannot be admitted, so the partial roots of prejudice are sown. Another root of prejudice is a need for the expression of aggression. Here the aggression is discharged on the hated–feared object, but what prejudiced person is aware of this?

The poor defenses always serve to reduce conscious ego function. They defend, but in the process they over-defend to the point where the ego functions even less well. People may be afraid of high places all their lives because of a long-repressed incident, or incidents, from their childhood. Here denial reduces a whole section of their world by causing intense anxiety in high places. They lose the ability to function in this situation by the continuance of an ego defense which, perhaps initially conscious and rational, now serves only to handicap. Any time a need, the world, or an ego function is denied, their loss hampers the ego in its job. This denial, never good, can at its worst be extremely handicapping, as in psychosis in which the use of denial is so massive that it extends to the point where the very existence of reality is blotted out.

Finally, a word about the emotions as they relate to the ego defenses. The emotions occur as ego reactions, not only to the conscious ego functions but also in exactly the same way as ego reactions to the ego defenses. Emotions occurring with sublimation are for the most part pleasant, whereas emotions occurring with the use of denial are primarily unpleasant. Emotions may also become unconscious by the use of denial. In depression, for example, the angry emotion is denied, and depression is experienced as a poor attempt at sublimation.

Appropriate or not, the conscious emotion, depression in the previous instance, is what we feel. We do not feel the ego defense which turned ego into depression. The ego defense is always either inadequate or unsatisfactory if we feel displeasure without any conscious reason.

Three things therefore are meant when we say a person is emotionally disturbed:

1. An unpleasant variety of emotions is experienced by this person, or by people around him because of him.
2. These emotions originate in the extensive use of poor or unsatisfactory ego defenses.
3. The ego defenses, in turn, have their origin in poor ego functioning, which is the basic cause.

6

Character or Personality—the Pattern of the Ego

CHARACTER OR PERSONALITY IS THE SUM TOTAL OF WHOLE ego operation. It includes the ego functions, the emotions or ego reactions, and the ego defenses. The character is the unique individual pattern which each ego develops to perform the three previous operations. The character that we see is often called the personality. We say a person is cold, warm, ineffective, violent, miserly, good or bad. These are partial descriptions of the over-all pattern of ego functioning, ego reactions, and the ego defenses. They cannot be separated, but are all united in a whole.

It is extremely difficult to describe the total pattern because in description there is a tendency to break the whole into component parts. The result of this fragmentation may be that the total impression of a personality is lost, for the parts are meaningless unless they are united into the whole, which is the personality. Often we are disappointed with psychological tests because they also tend to dissect personality, losing the flavor of the whole in the process. The results of these tests seem sparse compared to the many interwoven dimensions of the total personality to be evaluated. Only a few people, usually great writers, can describe personality in words. The ability to establish vividly the personality of the people they write about so we can feel the impact of this person's unique ego pattern is one of the marks of excellence of these writers.

We can compare the personality of an individual with an effective ego to a key, simple at first, and able to fit into only the largest, most general locks. As he grows older, more notches and ridges are cut into the key until it becomes a skeleton key able to open all previous locks, plus many new, intricate ones. Finally an extremely special key is developed, one which when placed in a strange lock is able both to fit itself to the lock and to open all but the most complex and difficult. Yet it retains both its basic shape and consistency and can easily be recognized as the original key. In this analogy the locks serve as the situations in the world with which the person learns to cope successfully as his personality (key) matures effectively. That no situation is ever identical to two people is the basic reason why no two personalities are ever the same. As previously stated, however, some people have ineffective ego functioning and, although they too have a pattern of functioning or a personality, it does not serve to make their egos more effective. The pattern may be too tight, or too loose, or both. It may be rigid and inflexible in some dimensions, completely unformed in others; a combination may exist. No two characters are exactly alike, but there are basic types of characters which accompany defective ego functioning.

An example of this type of character is the woman who has a passion for cleanliness, the "Craig's wife"[1] whose whole life is dominated by her cleanliness mania. This is her personality. All her ego functions are tempered by this compulsion. We say she has a "compulsive personality," her ego functions having bowed to this pattern. The situation can be likened to the dummy taking over the ventriloquist, the personality itself becoming a major ego defense. A compulsive individual always exhibits overwhelming anxiety when his personality is challenged by the world, as for example, a compulsively clean person might commit suicide if forced to live in dirt. Thus, the personality can do the person harm as well as good.

An individual with a mature personality defends himself in a way that does not interfere with effective ego functioning. He has a personality and an ego that are congruent. With a defective ego, the personality, if established, always hampers effective ego functioning because of fear. The ego overdefends, as did the Maginot Line in France which defended itself, but not the country. In the same way pathological characters defend themselves with little or no regard for the person to whom they are attached. They cut off the nose to spite the face, an old but applicable saying. The compulsive person may be clean to the point where he cannot use, much less enjoy, the things most important to him, a condition which developed from early defective ego functioning with extensive use of poor ego defenses, resulting in a defective personality. It is the job of the psychiatrist to work with the personality or character and in doing so aid all its components toward more effective functioning.

---

[1] G. E. Kelly, *Craig's Wife*—a play in which the title character sacrifices her marriage and her child because of her rigid compulsion toward order and cleanliness.

7

Development of the Ego

Heredity vs. Environment

IN THIS CHAPTER, WHICH DEALS WITH HOW THE EGO DEVELops from birth through maturity, it is necessary to ask one basic question before the discussion begins. This is the question of how much of the ego is heredity and how much develops by contact with the environment. Unfortunately this question cannot be answered now and it is doubtful whether it will ever be answered. If it cannot be answered, we must establish how important it is. Need we concern ourselves with it? In the overwhelming majority of cases we need not be concerned, because, as important as heredity may be in the development of the personality, nothing can be done about it. Aldous Huxley, in *Brave New World*,[1] outlined a future society where some influence on heredity can be exerted, although we are fortunately still a considerable distance from this "brave new world." Lysenko[2] and his theories are unacceptable to us, for we believe that in the processes of heredity change takes place slowly, affecting the human ego very little during any given period of time. Each person has intelligence to accomplish only so much, and attempts to train him further are doomed to failure.

Other people seem to be congenitally disposed toward psychotic ego functioning. Their ego structure is limited and set by heredity. There are very few people who seem congenitally disposed toward defective egos in comparison with

---

[1] Aldous Huxley, *Brave New World* (New York: Harper & Brothers, 1932).
[2] T. D. Lysenko, *Heredity and Its Variability*, New York: Columbia University Press, 1946). He postulates that the effect of environment could, within a short time, change hereditary characteristics; a theory much discredited outside the Soviet Union.

the vast number who function poorly with no provable heredity cause. In the past, heredity was sometimes blamed for defective ego functioning, but less stress is now placed on this cause. At one time it was thought that certain people, usually physically malformed, were born bad. They were often tortured and persecuted to the point where they had no chance for normal ego development. The insane were thought to be irreversibly defective, and even today epileptics carry the stigma of mental abnormality although there is usually no direct relationship between seizures and defective ego functioning. Classes or races of people are falsely believed to be inherently defective, or inferior to other classes.

The important thought derived from the above discussion is that each person is born with a unique inherent capacity to function. The extent to which a person fulfills his capacity is rarely limited by his potential. Very few people, if any, ever develop to the total extent of their ability, but the degree to which they do, as well as the speed and course which they take in this development, is primarily determined by their relationship with their environment.

Development of the Ego—The Baby

The first nine months of life are uncomplicated because they occur in the mother's womb, a world in which all immediate needs are adequately provided for. This world is consistent, and from what we have been able to learn, it is relatively comfortable. Although few data have yet been gathered on this subject, it seems safe to assume that in a normal, healthy mother, the unborn child has all his needs satisfied automatically. This situation is rudely and permanently interrupted with the occurrence of birth. Within the space of hours the newborn babe is catapulted into a world in which he cannot survive if left to his own initiative.

An examination of the newborn infant leads to several important observations. He is either crying or he is sleeping, alternating between these two states for twenty-four hours, when food is added to his world. Now when he cries, he is fed and then perhaps has a period of contented wakefulness before he goes back to sleep. Soon four basic patterns are established: (1) discomfort, (2) physiologic need satisfaction, (3) comfort, and (4) escape from reality or the world into sleep. These infantile patterns are approximately the same for almost all small children.

We must further examine the situation in terms of needs, ego functions, and ego reactions. The infant initially has strong, urgent physiologic needs along with rudiments of the other needs. In some form they are all there and must be satisfied. The baby does not have the ego function to satisfy his needs, but he does have the ability to exhibit strong, primitive ego reactions. He howls and thrashes until someone, usually his mother, responds to these reactions by filling his needs as well as she is able. In a sense the mother acts as if she were the infant's ego; actually she shares her developed ego with him so he may survive. The mother's ego now responds quickly to the child's ego reactions; when he howls or rages she jumps, but she also derives satisfaction when, his needs satisfied, he exhibits peace and contentment. Here is a situation where one ego, the mother's, is happily doing the work of two. She derives pleasure satisfying not her needs but those of the child. Also, in the relationship of the mother to child, the basis of love, an ingredient essential to ego development is defined. In these terms *love is sharing ego function and receiving warm feelings when this sharing provides need satisfaction along with pleasant feelings for someone else.*

It is important to understand that for the infant the world is the mother or mother substitute. In early infancy usually one person takes the major responsibility for each child. To the infant the world (i.e., the mother) is a total, loving place, which acts as his ego, satisfies his needs, and provides him with the resultant pleasure. Everything is fused: he has no ability to distinguish between his ego, his mother's ego, and the world as it exists around him. To the newborn baby they remain all the same for a period of months. At this early stage, the infant, developing little or no ego functioning of his own, begins to appreciate in a primitive, preconscious way that the borrowed ego functioning (his mother's) can make life more pleasant for him. Although it is not his ego, he is involved because his needs are being filled. He is now part of the process of staying alive, early beginning to sense that the situation in which this process is taking place is composed of himself and his mother. This realization, which occurs within the first two to four months after birth, is the beginning of ego functioning. It is the start of the process of identity (the awareness of I AM I, a person different from my mother), as well as the beginning of the function of judgment in the dim realization that something is going on in which he, the infant, is taking part.

Development of the Ego—Theoretical Considerations

Immediately after birth, the mother's ego functions for the infant, deriving both happiness and satisfaction from this state of affairs. Sooner or later, however, there comes a time when the mother withdraws some of her ego functioning from the child. This process occurs gradually during the whole of childhood. Its initiation, however, is a crucial step. How and when the mother allows the child's ego to take over in its own right is the most important milestone in the development of an effective ego in the child. Although there are countless ways in which this can be done, here we are concerned with what is basically the right way.

The process, which should begin early if the child is going to develop an effective ego, must start long before the child can actually take over his own functioning. Consider, for example, a child two to four months old. He can do little with his primitive ego except howl. Although his ego cannot function very well, it can react so that he protests mightily when he feels lack of need satisfaction. Mother, at this critical time, has two choices. Following one alternative, she can take care of him properly, according to what is good, accepted physical care. If he still is not satisfied, however, she should let him howl. Allowed to remain in an uncomfortable situation, he can do little or nothing about it. If, following the second alternative, the mother is galvanized into nervous action because she cannot bear to hear the child cry, he will miss the beginning of normal ego development. Learning to react with bad feelings and anger to someone else's ego, he will miss the first step in the development of an effective ego, the realization that only so much will be done for him. He will also miss the beginning of the two-way relationship between himself and his mother. Early, of course, the relationship was necessarily one way, with Mother providing everything and baby accepting her offerings, protesting only when they were not enough. Now when he protests, Mother, having done everything necessary, lets him howl, in direct opposition to a widely taught misconception that babies should be ministered to on "demand." Soon he learns, even at the age of a few months, in spite of his crying, that nothing more will be done, and that his ego reactions, forceful as they are, are not producing the usual effect in his mother. Probably thinking about this for awhile in his primitive way, he soon decides to go to sleep. Sleep lets him escape from his discomfort and also solves the basic problem, fatigue. He is learning that he has to accept the fact that his mother's ego will continue to function for him most of the time, but not all of the time. Some of the time it is up to him, even if he only goes to sleep.

Let us examine this series of events from the mother's viewpoint. In the beginning she readily accepts the fact that she must function for her baby and that she loves him and enjoys doing it. Soon, however, Baby begins to be hard work. Even for the mother who has the maximum of love there are times when she does not feel like functioning for him. Sometimes she has other responsibilities and/or she feels like doing something for herself, possibly resting or sleeping. At these times Baby's crying irritates her to the point where, if she is honest, she wishes he would be still. At

DEVELOPMENT OF THE EGO

this time, early in the baby's career, a good mother makes the crucial decision. She decides, "I love my baby and I take good care of him, but I have my own needs too, so when he is fed and as comfortable as I can make him, I will leave him alone and take a rest myself."

This mother helps the child in his development by setting up a situation for future effective ego functioning. She shows him early in life that he exists in the world; at the same time she lets him know that the world is not set up expressly to satisfy his needs. That is, she teaches him that he is a part of the world instead of the world being a part of him. She finds it easy to take care of him because she respects herself and her own needs; she is not a slave to his ego reactions. Thus, a two-way relationship develops early in life, each person respecting both himself and the other person. The child is able to use his own ego in small ways to entertain himself, to see what he can do in the world. Early he begins to realize that in some ways he can achieve something with his own ego. His mother then is relieved for a little time of the responsibility of providing for all his needs. She pauses in her activity, deriving great satisfaction in what he can do for himself. While she lets him do certain things for himself, she still protects him from danger.

In the case described the mother and child have developed a good two-way relationship. The child, not totally dependent on the mother, from a very early age has been left to his own devices after all that is necessary has been done for him. She, in turn, does not feel guilty or less of a mother because she does not respond with military fervor to every whimper. She enjoys seeing her child develop independently as her relationship to him evolves. The mother sets the pattern for the child's ego function by trying him in situations where his ego must take over. He learns ego functioning primarily from his mother but also by himself. Enjoying the love of his mother, he can use it as an incentive for his own development rather than as a means of forcing his mother into doing things he should learn to do for himself.

The final important point in this relationship is that hostility or anger is minimal. No one can completely subordinate his own needs to those of someone else, not even a mother to a child, without feeling some anger. If the proper two-way relationship exists, this anger is minimized, and the child matures with an effective ego. If, however, the mother attempts to respond to all of her child's protests of discomfort, she becomes angry, and, even though she continues to care for him, the anger she feels is communicated to the child. Unable to handle hostility—only a well-developed, effective ego can handle hostility, and in such a situation there is little if any ego development—the child is terrified by the paradox which now exists. Although he has his needs satisfied with his mother's ego functioning for him, he feels her anger. The fear generated by the mother's anger completely immobilizes the infant so that he is afraid to go further, the anger stopping his progress in its tracks. He needs to develop his ego from the pattern set by his mother, but he cannot do so because her anger blocks him. He reacts by becoming terrified and screaming, with the unfortunate result that she gets angrier. The mother-child relationship, so important to the child's ego growth, may deteriorate, so that neither gains satisfaction. She must do more and more for him with her ego, thus compounding the situation which started her original anger.

Two important concepts can now be delineated. *First, ego growth cannot take place in the presence of anger unless the ego is strong enough to handle the situation without fear.* Thus punishment of ego-defective delinquents never works; the only solution is to help their egos to grow in an atmosphere of consistency and acceptance. *Second, it is important to develop relationships which are two-way, with each person respecting the other and each deriving satisfaction from seeing the other person fill his own needs.* These two concepts are the basis of all ego growth and, as will be explained later, they, with certain additions, are the basis of psychotherapy.

DEVELOPMENT OF THE EGO

The child who has learned to develop a good two-way relationship with his mother is ready to progress rapidly in life, further developing an effective ego. He develops the same type of relationship with his father, sisters, brothers, relatives, friends and schoolteachers. He gives as well as takes, as he finds that few people are hostile to him. In the relationships with these people his ego grows rapidly. He can take from them what he needs because it is given willingly. He learns to feel, to think, to judge, and to develop values by relating to many people. Because each person respects him as an individual, he gains early a strong sense of I AM I, which continues to grow, so that he feels comfortable in his own unique identity. When he encounters stressful situations, he either has the ego strength to handle them or he knows where to go for protection. In his development those who love him guide him toward independence, but as they do so they adhere to one main principle—they help avoid situations which demand more ego strength than the child has at the time.

As an example, a good father should not demand that his young son be a star baseball player. Accepting the child's limitations, he does not show anger or resentment when his son strikes out in a crucial inning in a Little League game. Again, a child who is allowed to cross a quiet street at five years of age, and who is taught the danger of traffic when he is old enough to understand, is properly protected from those dangers that he cannot comprehend. Also, the small child should not be subjected to motion pictures, TV, or "comic" books so violent that his immature ego, unable to cope with the emotions aroused, produces fear which in turn retards his emotional development. He should not, however, be overprotected or kept from breaking all rules. He must learn to take responsibility for his own actions early. The proper balance is a matter of parental judgment.

Later in life, if a correct start has been made, effective ego development continues at an ever-increasing rate. The growing person makes more relationships, enriching his ego functions from them. Unafraid of people or situations, he even profits from emotional stresses and acute frustrations. He learns and matures, not only from relating to people, but also he develops the ability to grow from abstract media such as books, plays, music, and ideas. They all become meaningful as they filter into his growing ego. Thus the individual develops an effective ego, which in turn provides him with the ultimate reward any human can expect, the chance to realize fully his inherent mental capacities.

Development of the Ego—Some Practical Considerations

The ideal pattern for effective ego development has been explained. There are, however, many people with effective egos who did not follow the pattern laid out. It is necessary to understand that, from a practical standpoint, if one important criterion has been fulfilled it is possible to produce an effective ego.

This criterion states that: *To develop an effective ego, a person must have a meaningful, two-way relationship with someone who has an effective ego—a relationship in which the ego of the giving person is available for use by the receiving person in a consistent atmosphere of some love and a minimum of hostility or anger.*

This means, in simple words, that in order to develop an effective ego we must in most cases be exposed to at least one person with an effective ego who cares about us. The earlier this occurs in life the better; in the ideal case it is first the mother, then the father, and after that almost everyone. Practically, this situation rarely exists in exactly the ideal way, with the result that few of us are fortunate enough to develop an effective ego early in life. Most of us develop an effective ego sometime after early childhood, and a few people do so only late in life, perhaps even as they approach death, as in the case of people who have their first good relationship with a doctor or nursing attendant in a final fatal disease. An example in literature is Sydney Carton, in *A Tale of Two Cities*,[3] although we can only speculate about why his ego suddenly grew so effective.

To repeat, we must have at least one good relationship, hopefully more than one, but the minimum is one. Thus, it would seem that if we have the misfortune to relate only to people with varying degrees of defective ego function, we would have no chance for establishing good ego functions. There are rare exceptions, however, because the human ego, as it develops, is sometimes able to derive benefit from relationships with various people who have less than effective egos. Because no one has a completely defective ego, each person is able to give something good to the person with the developing ego. In these rare cases many partially defective egos can be pooled by the person in his growth toward an effective ego, with the result that he may fashion a fairly effective ego for himself out of a group of egos effective only in part.

Other factors affecting ego development are the relative ego strength and the sex of the giver. A person with an effective ego can give more, so that one relationship with such a person is worth many relationships with people with less effective egos. The sex of the giving person probably makes some difference in establishing identity. The earlier one has a good relationship with a person of the same sex, the more easily the basic ego function of sexual identity is established. Once this is done, the sex of the giver makes little difference in the development of an effective ego.

We wonder why people from good social backgrounds with "advantages" sometimes develop poor ego functioning. This can be explained in terms of the relationships which they had earlier or later in life. We can postulate that either or both of two things must have happened: (1) Although they were exposed to people with good func-

[3] Charles Dickens: *A Tale of Two Cities* in which Sydney Carton, a ne'er-do-well, finds enough ego strength to sacrifice his life for a worthwhile person.

tioning, no two-way relationship was formed, or (2) the people with whom they did relate had defective egos.

Thus, despite the opportunity, something went awry.

Equally puzzling is the question of why two boys coming from the same slum area rise to such different heights. One may become a social success, while the other ends up behind bars. We cannot explain how such great differences can occur even between brothers if we do not understand that in one case the criterion was met while in the other case it was not.

From the above discussion it may be seen that a person's obvious background, as it is revealed in much ordinary personal history, is of little or no importance. Similarly evident is the huge waste of time and money being expended fruitlessly in psychological and sociological research programs which employ tests and forms. No matter how much data is gleaned in this manner it is rarely of value because it reflects poorly the exact interpersonal relationships which are the crux of ego development. Although information on the exact relationships is subjective and difficult to obtain, it is the data of real importance in case histories.

In some instances relationships with people with defective egos produce other defective egos. If the person with whom the developing ego relates has a specific type of ego defect, it may be transferred directly. Examples of this process are common, the most usual being the fears, superstitions, and prejudices of the parents that are often transferred to the child. This occurs because the parent has a defective ego and, if no one else intervenes, the child is left with similarly poor functioning. Thus some defective ego functioning is perpetuated through families. We all know families so afflicted, and it is easy to predict what people in them will be like because they develop a defective pattern, a defective family personality. This pattern does not change unless, by stroke of fortune, someone with an effective ego moves into the family, a rare situation because people with effective egos stay away from them. A recent admission to a school for delinquent girls told the interviewer that her mother was in jail, her father just out on parole, both brothers were in a reformatory, and she had three uncles in San Quentin. There is little chance to develop an effective ego in such a family.

Finally, and outwardly quite confusing, is the situation in which people, willing or not, may be the tools of other people's egos. Here we must examine some other aspects of conscious and unconscious behavior. To a great extent relationships between people take place at a level of which neither is consciously aware. Sometimes, for reasons far from apparent, people "instinctively" dislike each other, whereas, to cite an opposite example, love at first sight is a strong positive attraction between two people which defies rational explanation. Forces operate to which both egos respond, but which at least in the beginning are not clear to either. Although the attraction or repulsion factor in the relationship may eventually become clear, in many cases it never does. Often there is no desire on the part of either person to explore these factors because they are satisfied with the status quo.

In some cases, however, unconscious factors may be involved in ego development to the extent that serious difficulty ensues. This situation exists when the ego of the giver is unable, for various reasons, to fill certain of his own needs, or to react in some ways because of certain bad ego defenses—defenses which lead to a character without a pattern to fill these needs. The unfilled needs may be transmitted to the receiver so that although they are not his own unfulfilled needs, due to the relationship he may feel as if they were. This transmission, which I called borrowed ego functioning, may take place at a level not conscious to either.

For example: a mother may be sexually frustrated, unable to fulfill her own strong sexual needs. She cannot successfully sublimate these needs, nor can she deny them without feeling strong anxiety and discomfort. If she has a daughter, however, she may transmit to her, at a level beneath the daughter's awareness, the fact that she cannot fulfill her own needs. She also transmits the thought, "If you, my daughter, will fulfill these needs for me, I will be happy," in much the same way that she might transmit the thought that if the daughter did well in school she would be happy. The sexual needs, however, pose a problem. Satisfying them is far different from the need for daughter to do well in school, because consciously the mother says, "Be good, and lead a respectable sexual life like me," while unconsciously the mother transmits, "Go ahead and have sexual relations so that I can enjoy them vicariously, which for me will be better than my present sex life." To both daughter and mother this may become a confusing, even tragic, state of affairs.

Along with the unconscious transmission of this need is the further admonition, "If you, daughter, do not do this, I will withdraw my love," whereas consciously the reverse is stated. In these situations the unconscious motivation usually is stronger, probably because it is the true motivation. The daughter has been forced to borrow a part of the mother's ego which then impels her to behave, not from her own needs but from the mother's. She furnishes the body, the mother the ego. If she rejects this borrowed ego, the mother will withdraw the love which the daughter needs so badly. The daughter may then indulge in a series of sexual acts which, horrifying both the mother and daughter on a conscious level, fulfill their unconscious contract. Although this behavior may stop if the mother's vicarious satisfactions are sufficient, it sometimes leads to much conscious hostility between them—hostility that is always extremely upsetting to them both as well as baffling to the social authorities who become involved if the child is underage. The above example is only one of many possible variations of borrowed ego functioning. It is often the only explanation for acts by people who ordinarily are horrified even to read about such behavior. Borrowed ego functioning is further discussed under incomplete ego functioning in Chapter 8.

In some cases borrowed ego functioning may benefit the recipient. For example, parents who are ignorant to the point of consciously extolling the virtues of ignorance may unconsciously communicate the virtues of education to their children, although they may never be really comfortable in the presence of the educated offspring. They have lent a portion of their ego which has done much for the child.

In conclusion it must be stated that any and all combinations of all the types of ego development may occur. They may occur in any time sequence or concurrently. It is this infinity of variations which leads to the development of unique personalities, some developing haphazardly, some strong and purposefully developed, and some in various other states of development. One sad but remarkable aspect of ego development is that out of all the possible combinations so many similar personalities exist. This lack of variation is the mark of a culture which has fallen into set patterns, a world, which, for all its complexities, is without much variety for many individuals, an organized society which makes life difficult for people who wish to express the uniqueness of personality inherent in man.

II

ABNORMAL HUMAN FUNCTIONING

Introduction

In recent years there has been much discussion in schools of all levels about abnormal human functioning, ranging from beginning courses in "'Abnormal Psych" offered in the sophomore year in college to advanced seminars on abnormal psychopathology which are requisites in the training of a psychoanalyst. Schools of psychology vie with one another in efforts to explain those wide variations in functioning which are labeled abnormal. The disciplines of psychology, psychiatry, sociology, anthropology, and philosophy are ever concerned with this aspect of human functioning. Both old and modern legends, plays, and literature abound with examples of abnormal psychology, from *Oedipus Rex* through *Hamlet* to the tortured Blanche Dubois in Tennessee Williams' *A Street Car Named Desire*. Every type of deviant human behavior has been richly chronicled in literature, often more accurately than in scientific works.

In this part an effort is made to explain psychopathology in terms of various types of defective egos. Full descriptions of aberrant behavior are not presented, as they are adequately described in many available popular psychiatric texts. Rather, an attempt is made to tie together the familiar classes of abnormal behavior and to explain why people with these types of defective egos behave the way they do.

The regular diagnostic terms used in psychiatry will be correlated with ego functioning, although no brief is held for the use of these terms. They are used because they have become a part of the language, although for a clear understanding of abnormal behavior they leave much to be desired. It is hoped that eventually these present diagnostic terms will be replaced by descriptive terms based on the type of defective ego which predominates in that class of abnormality.

The various types of defective egos are described in this section as separate entities because they are most easily perceived in that way. In many cases they do occur as distinct conditions but this is not always so. There is no psychological law that a person must have a particular type of ego defect to the exclusion of others. Most people, even those with effective egos, have many different types of ego defects. We are all at times a little neurotic, a little psychotic, and have elements of character disorder and depression. Few of us escape some manifestation of psychosomatic disease at one time or another.

We have these ego defects transiently as our ego is constantly adjusting to variations of internal and external stresses. People with defective egos rarely have rigidly fixed defects. In some cases they alternate from one defect to another, sometimes even quite regularly as, for example, a person who alternates between depression and psychosomatic disease. Because people can have more than one serious ego defect at the same time and the defects can change, there is rarely a fixed pattern which can be counted on. The whole ego is in a constant state of flux, always seeking different ways to do its job. In most patients, however, one type of ego defect predominates, and it is by this predominant defect that abnormal functioning is classified. When reading this part do not be disappointed if people you know can't be made to fit into any category, or surprised if some others fit remarkably well.

8

Incomplete Ego Functioning—Personality or Character Disorders

MANY PEOPLE IN OUR SOCIETY ARE UNABLE TO FOLLOW the accepted rules and laws. Suffering from a personality or character disorder, they act as though law and social order did not exist although paradoxically they know they are doing wrong. These offenders, who include almost all juvenile lawbreakers and many adult criminals, are powerless to stop their antisocial behavior. Unless fortunate, protected by money or influence, or killed in some dangerous pursuit, they sooner or later run afoul of the law. At this point society asks: What's wrong with these people, why can't they follow the rules? Why do they feel little or no remorse for their actions? Why are they so hostile? So destructive? Why are they so impervious to help? What can be done? Who can help them? These are legitimate questions, and it is the obligation of the psychiatrist to attempt to answer them.

The most important question is: What is wrong with these people? or, Why is a juvenile delinquent delinquent? Following the principles discussed in Part I it is the author's opinion that this large group of people have incomplete egos. This means that their egos are not completely formed even though they may have reached physical maturity. In terms of the diagram in Chapter 3, they have holes or gaps or incomplete areas in their egos.

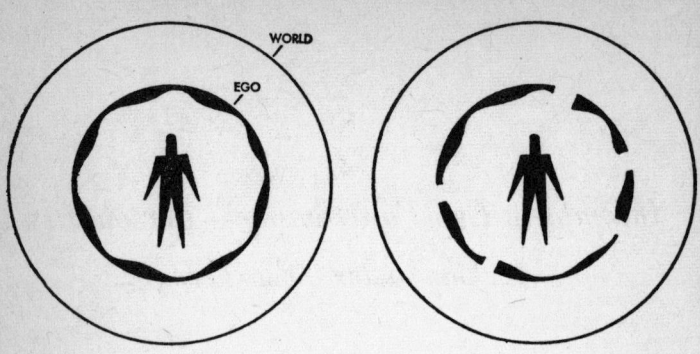

The illustration at the left shows the normal ego which completely surrounds the person and is at all times mediating and contacting all areas in the world. This normal ego functions to fill the needs and protect the person within the rules of the world. The juvenile delinquent, or person with a character disorder, suffers from incomplete ego development with the result that his ego does not form a complete protective, functioning circle around him. Instead it is full of gaps, it is incomplete. The ego has gaps because it never was completely formed. A person with such an ego has the serious problem of trying to function in the world with a defective ego, defective in the respect that it is incomplete.

The ego may have only one small gap, or it may be so shot with holes that it is virtually nonexistent. This variation can be illustrated by the following diagrams:

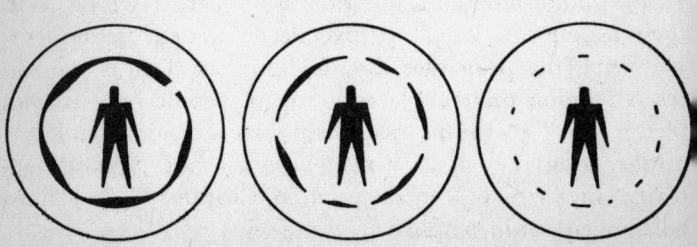

INCOMPLETE EGO FUNCTIONING

The situation, however, is not as simple as these diagrams would seem to indicate because the ego is never static. Gaps in the ego can open and close as well as shift position. It is this shifting which explains the erratic and unpredictable behavior of people with character disorders—there are always gaps but where at one time there is ego the next time there may be none.

Continuing this line of reasoning to answer the original questions on the behavior of the juvenile delinquent, the next logical question is: How do these gaps affect his functioning? If one does not have a complete ego, several detrimental events will occur.

First and most important is that to have effective ego functioning one must have a strong sense of I AM I. A person who has a fragmented ego can never have this feeling. He doesn't have a conviction of personal identity; he doesn't know who he is. With his limited ego he can feel only empty and shattered. Isolated sections of his ego may fleetingly experience different identities. Due to his lack of continuity he may at times feel that he is two or three different people, although usually he feels that he is no one at all. He never senses strongly who he is even if he does feel a weak or transient identity. In his confusion he may shift from one identity to another in an effort to find one which may relieve for a time the painful sensation of emptiness.

The second important consequence of an incomplete ego is that the person necessarily has defective judgment. This causes difficulty because he is unable to obey the rules and regulations necessary to get along in society. Usually he has enough ego so that he vaguely knows the rules, but he can't apply them. To illustrate: Imagine a person with a hole in his ego—just one gap, one area where there is no ego function.

This is a person who in many situations can get along all right. He can exercise judgment in all areas except in the space covered by the gap in his ego. If he has to fill a need according to Arrow 1, the need is felt by his intact,

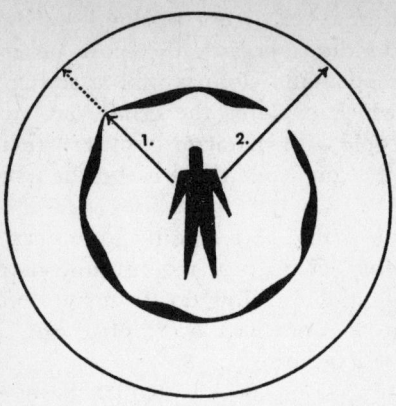

functioning ego and is mediated according to the rules. Not so the need designated by Arrow 2. Here a need travels directly out to the world, unmediated by ego function. The person acts as though there were no rules or regulations in the fulfillment of this need. The need, unmodified by the ego, contacts the world with all its primitive force.

Suppose the need is sexual, and it goes out unmodified. In this case the person may commit an act of rape to satisfy the need. He may act without feeling, judgment, or awareness of the consequences. He may dimly sense that he is acting wrong, but he will be powerless to stop the activity because no ego is involved. The primitive need is acted upon as though society and its rules did not exist, because for these rules to be meaningful they must exist within ourselves as a part of the ego. The person committing rape is in serious difficulty because he lacked the judgment to mediate his sexual need properly. It must be understood that while the need may be filled, the rapist gets little satisfaction since the feeling of satisfaction is in the ego, not in the act. Thus the rapist with this type of defective ego may senselessly repeat his behavior. He is only stopped by external control—police action and incarceration.

When the ego is incomplete further detrimental consequences may follow. As explained previously, the ego is not only the mechanism which mediates and satisfies needs, it also protects the person from dangers in the world. If a person has gaps in his ego, he is defenseless against anything in the world which may come through those gaps.

Juveniles play a game they call Chicken—one dares another to do a dangerous or foolhardy act. The child who accepts the challenge has no judgment, no ability to say No. The external challenge comes through a gap and he takes the dare, often suffering serious consequences. Later he can't understand why he did it, but if he is "fortunate" enough to get another chance he may repeat the experience over and over. The function of identity is also operating here. The child takes the dare in an attempt to establish a desirable identity in the eyes of his companions because he did not have the feeling of I AM I which accompanies an intact ego.

A person with gaps in his ego has none of the rich emotional feelings intrinsic to good ego functioning. His ego reactions are anger and emptiness: anger because he is frustrated in his attempts to fill his needs satisfactorily, and emptiness because he has no real sense of identity. He operates psychologically with these gaps just as a man who has an organic defect operates physically. He is handicapped psychologically in the same way that a prize fighter with a broken hand is handicapped physically. While he sees other people filling their needs, he can't fill his, nor can he protect himself from ordinary dangers in the world if they come through a gap in his ego so that he has no choice but to be continually frustrated and angry. Miserable because he is "filled" with emptiness, he grows to hate, expressing his anger at those who get along. He destroys property which exemplifies those things which he doesn't have or which stands for the rules of society. A favorite object of juvenile destruction is a public school, which stands as a symbol of social order and progress, values in which he is grossly deficient.

Feeling inferior and incomplete in the presence of people with effective egos who in most cases do not want him, he tends to group himself with a gang of people like himself. Thus, his defect isolates him from those who could help him; the delinquent and his society become separated from our society by fear and anger on both sides. Although his peers give him no true satisfaction, at least they are not frightened of him, and they have the same troubles and confusions that he has. In his gang he feels more protected and is better able to express his hostile feelings. Another reason for joining the gang is to obtain some sense of identity, wherein he uses other gang members partly to piece in the gaps in his ego, but, in the same process, he surrenders part of his ego to the group. The gang, standing as a complete, hostile, angry, destructive group ego with which he can identify, thus relieves some of his emptiness. This group identity needs constant reinforcement, only functioning well when it is destroying property or showing its superiority to other gangs in street fights. As a gang member he may fight viciously and even kill because he does not have enough effective ego to control his anger or to appreciate the significance of his acts until it is too late.

In an effort to gain a sense of identity he may purposefully get into difficulty over and over, often repeating the same acts. He does this to establish his identity by getting caught and going through a legal process where police will literally or figuratively beat him so that he feels that he exists. He is also caught because he may have enough ego function to realize that unless he is controlled externally by the law he will destroy himself. He settles for external control so that he may feel a little peace from the helplessness caused by his ego defect.

Although a person with a character disorder has no good inner feelings, no positive, warm ego reactions, he still needs satisfactions. Unable to find them within himself, he is dependent on external "kicks." He listens eagerly to every story of how someone else got satisfaction. For normal satisfactions we use our egos, as it is in our egos that we feel; the person with a character disorder, however, has little feeling because his ego is full of gaps. He gets his satisfying experiences in a primitive way by actual physical feelings. Always looking for physical stimulation, or "kicks," as he puts it, he will take dope, smoke marijuana, and drink almost anything despite the danger to his health. For example, in a typical school for adolescent delinquent girls there are less than 10 per cent who have not smoked marijuana.

Another characteristic of this type of ego defect is an aberrant sexual life. The juvenile delinquent indulges in excessive sexual play early, often engaging extensively in sexual intercourse although in most cases he obtains little or no satisfaction. Sexual intercourse is often regarded as an aggressive act, so that he has no feeling for his partner; this lack of feeling is usually reciprocated as the partner he finds usually has the same ego defect. Soon finding sex no better than masturbation, he is unable to understand people who talk of love and tenderness. Girls, especially puzzled by the lack of fulfillment in this widely ballyhooed experience, may turn to pseudo-homosexuality in an effort to find sexual expression. This is not the true homosexuality to be discussed later, but rather a turning away from the brutality of heterosexuality as the girl has experienced it.

In severe cases of fragmented ego functioning, drug addiction may occur. Drug addicts are always people with markedly incomplete ego functioning. Feeling the anger and emptiness caused by their lack of ego, they may turn to the opiate drugs. These drugs, of which heroin is the most common, appear to fill a definite place in their lives. Heroin acts for the addict as a panacea for his difficulties. It is almost a specific for his ego problems, for it seems to fill the gaps in his ego. The addict tells you that when he is "high" he feels no emptiness, no anger, only a deep feeling of satisfaction. For heroin addicts it is often the first time in their lives they have had a feeling of well-being, so that, besides its known physiologic effect, the drug produces a deep-seated psychological addiction.

Without this drug the person looks forward to a life with no peace, only emptiness and anger, which to him is an intolerable existence once he has experienced the contentment produced by heroin in his blood. Actively proselyting his addiction with the same fervor as a man trying to convert others to a new-found "true" religion, in many cases he attempts to start others on the drug. He may do this because he feels he is doing them a favor or, more often, for the purpose of selling them drugs to obtain money for his own habit. If he is deprived of drugs he will often become so desperate that he will beg, borrow, steal and sometimes even murder for a "fix." He can't be persuaded with logic that heroin is a deadly drug because, as he blandly and truthfully says, without the drug he would rather be dead.

People who have incomplete egos are always prey for heroin addiction, whereas people with effective egos almost never become addicted. They may do so under unusual circumstances where their effective ego was under great stress as, for example, in people who have been severely injured and need long periods of narcotics for relief of physical pain. Most people with effective egos, however, do not like the feeling produced by narcotics and under ordinary conditions it is almost impossible for them to become addicts.

Prominent in the person with the character disorder is a remarkable lack of anxiety. They feel emptiness and anger but very little anxiety. Previously it was stated that the purpose of anxiety is to warn the ego that it is failing in its function. Although this anxiety mechanism works in most people, even those who have moderately defective egos, it does not work with character disorders because they rarely have enough functioning ego to feel anxiety. Thus they go on their way without this powerful built-in warning system operating. They are bland and noncommittal even when charged with serious crimes, quickly adopting the two pathologic defenses, projection and denial. In shootings they say, "It was the other guy's fault because he pulled a gun." In car thefts where the car is wrecked, they say, "What's the difference? The car was insured." Using any number of evasions or denials with no concern, these people seem incapable of feeling. Unless we understand that they do not have sufficient ego structure to feel anxiety, this lack is extremely puzzling. When they start to feel anxiety and, even better, responsibility for their actions, they are no longer personality disorders.

The final question then presents itself when we ask: How do people get this way? Under what circumstances do people grow to physical maturity with such large gaps in their egos? Let us briefly re-examine how an effective ego develops. It was pointed out that the minimal criterion for an effective ego is that the person must have a good two-way relationship with someone with an effective ego who cares for him. Although it might seem that this type of relationship would be available to everyone, unfortunately it is not. Children grow up without ever having had even the beginnings of development in association with someone who cares and who can help them establish a two-way relationship. In a typical school for delinquent girls less than 5 per cent come from an intact home, and even of this 5 per cent the home, while intact, is far from able to provide the minimal criterion for good ego development. People have children regardless of the state of their own egos and their ability to transmit effective ego functioning. Unless the child at an early age can develop the ability to engage in two-way relationships, most people outside his home won't care enough to relate to him, thus early isolating him from society and forcing him into groups of his peers. As previously mentioned, only in rare instances can effective egos develop with a variety of poor relationships early in life.

Unable to develop minimal early relationships, the child grows into adolescence and maturity with the body and needs corresponding to his chronological age, but with a fragmented ego. Although parts of the ego are intact, they in no way form a complete, flexible, effective functioning ego. When the child operates through the intact parts, or when he is externally controlled, as he can be when preadolescent, he gets along in society, but eventually he gets out of control. Parents, often horrified by the results when their child gets into trouble, attempt drastic measures to control him. Usually this is too late, because love is lacking and fear and anger are predominant. This is not the climate for good ego growth, and the gaps remain unfilled.

This chapter discusses primarily those people who have gross defects in their egos. They have fragmented egos which can't begin to cope with the world and its rules or with their own strong needs. While the majority of people with character disorders are able to stay out of corrective or penal institutions, there are enough who come into conflict with the law to comprise a large percentage of those persons committed.

Another large group, labeled personality disorders, have what can be described as borrowed ego functioning. Their own egos are incomplete, but in combination with the "donor" or lender their ego is relatively intact. These are extremely dependent people who, unable to shift for themselves, are so "other directed" that they need the other person's ego all the time and are lost when removed from the donor. They have not developed enough ego of their own to function, and the donor has neither the proper relationship nor the desire to set them free. For example, these are the sons and daughters who never leave home and mother, and the henpecked husbands who can't stand alone. Although recognizing and even rebelling against their dependent situation, these people are powerless to do anything about it. They can't leave this position because they know that they are helpless without the borrowed part of the ego. In many cases they take alcohol to escape from the hopelessness of their position either while in their dependent status or after the donor passes away. The alcohol acting as anesthesia helps them by serving as a partial substitute for active effective ego, something they desire but never have. These people, in a sense enslaved by their peculiar position, are extremely hard to help because the borrowed ego serves as a block to prevent ego growth. At the same time that it fills the gaps, it prevents them from closing.

It is also a Trilby-Svengali relationship in most cases. The donor gets some satisfaction from the helplessness of the borrower because he can sometimes use this person as a tool for needs which he himself is unable to fulfill. In the case of the sexually acting-out daughter described in Chapter 7, the actual ego mechanism may now be understood. In this type of ego functioning, the daughter, acting out promiscuously, is using a borrowed part of her mother's ego and, in a sense, the mother's donated ego is using her daughter's body. Operating consciously or unconsciously, this mechanism is the cause of many delinquent acts in people of both sexes and all ages. Only when the chain is broken in some way can help be given to the borrower, the Trilby.

Sometimes these people, using anger generated through parts of their own ego, turn on the donor and destroy him as, for example, in cases of children attacking or killing a "beloved" mother. By committing such an act, however, they are left with their own ego almost totally fragmented so that they are extremely difficult to help psychiatrically. The treatment of these as well as the other character disorders is discussed in Part III of this book.

9

Ego Weakness—Neurotic Ego Functioning— Neuroses

NEUROSIS OR EGO WEAKNESS IS THE MOST COMMON FORM of ego defect. In terms of the previously used circle diagrams, neurosis may be represented as follows:

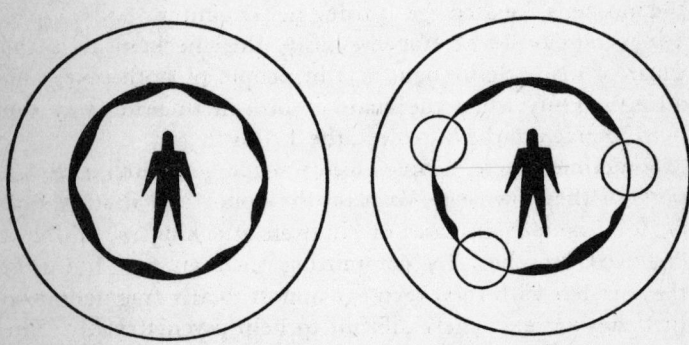

NORMAL OR EFFECTIVE EGO   **NEUROTIC EGO**

Circled areas in the neurotic ego are areas of ego weakness. In distinction from the character disorders, the ego is complete but does not have the strong, flexible continuity found in the effective ego.

Ego weakness may be confined to specific areas of the ego as in the above diagram of the neurotic ego. In these cases there develops what is termed a symptom neurosis, that is, a neurosis in which there is a specific symptom. In other cases the ego weakness may be generalized to include the whole ego. This may be diagramed as follows:

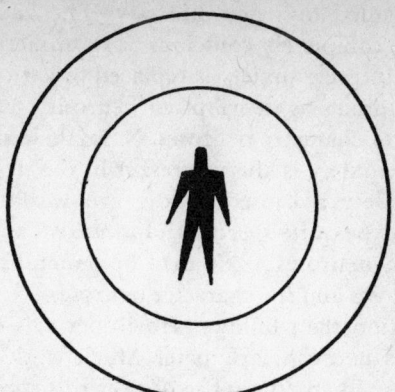

The whole ego is weak, though it is
still complete.

The cases where the ego weakness is generalized are the anxiety neuroses, the character neuroses, and the sexual neuroses. In the following chapters these various forms of the neuroses will be discussed in detail.

Neurosis is so common among psychologically sophisticated people that to call oneself neurotic conjures up more humor than derogation. Because no one is completely free from ego weakness, it is the amount of this type of ego defect which in part defines the condition. A small amount of ego weakness does little to hamper effective ego functioning; neurosis, however, occurs when the ego weakness reaches a point where ego functioning is impaired. In most cases neurosis is obvious to the patient or to someone observing his functioning, because the neurotic person handles anxiety in a pathological way. As will be explained later, the neurotic person has a defect in his ego which makes it impossible for him to cope with anxiety effectively.

The neurotic person always develops pathological ways to avoid anxiety. Thus the essence of neurosis is an ego weakness plus an inability to handle anxiety effectively. Although anxiety exists in all people to varying degrees, in neurosis it is always handled in a neurotic way. The anxiety in some cases may be completely conscious as in anxiety neurosis; in most cases, however, anxiety is replaced to various degrees by neurotic symptoms as in symptom neurosis or by a neurotic character as in character neuroses. Nevertheless, conscious or unconscious anxiety is always present in the neurotic process and this anxiety is caused by the ego weakness. The ego weakness may be quite *specific* and *localized*, as in the case of the symptom neuroses, or it may be *generalized*, as in the anxiety neuroses and the character neuroses.

The question then follows: How does this ego weakness, which causes neurosis, originate? Much work in psychiatry has been done in an attempt to answer this specific question. Although many elaborate theoretical formulations have been advanced, there is one crucial aspect of this process which, though relatively simple, is probably of prime importance. This is the atmosphere in which the neurotic person is raised. As previously stated the basis of neurosis is an ego weakness leading to anxiety. The anxiety, however, would not necessarily cause neurotic ego functioning; it is how the person handles the anxiety that is crucial to the process. In examining neurotic people it can be seen that they all have a deep and inordinate fear of anxiety. There is something defective in their ego which leads them to feel that they cannot handle anxiety. They feel compelled to try to rid themselves of it at all costs. That the neurosis compounds this difficulty they do not understand.

Because they are unable to accept anxiety they not only strive mightily to avoid it themselves, but also (1) attempt to create a situation for their children in which there is little or no anxiety, or (2) try to relieve their anxiety by transferring it to their children, often burdening the child with anxiety that his immature ego cannot yet handle. In some cases, incongruous as it may seem, both of these conditions may occur simultaneously or alternately.

These then are the principal conditions for the production of neurosis. If this line of reasoning is accepted, it follows that neurosis breeds neurosis. In distinction from the character disorders, which occur haphazardly due to the lack of any relationship, neurosis is bred in the presence of a definite but neurotic relationship. The relationship exists between the child who is later to have a neurosis and some of the important people to whom he relates in his development. Not all neurotic parents, however, produce neurotic children. In some cases children may form good relationships with people other than their parents who make up for the parental ego weakness, and in others parents may recognize their neuroses so that although they may be able to do little to help themselves, they *are* able to avoid neurotic interaction with their children.

The process is initiated, in most cases, by a parent who has an excessive fear of anxiety. He may take the first of the two courses described above by doing his utmost to protect his child from feeling anxiety. He does so because he feels it is important to protect his child against what he, the parent, fears most—anxiety. Parents falsely believe that if they protect their child from experiencing anxiety when young, as he grows older and "stronger" he *will* be able to cope with it. Ten to thirty years ago this belief was shared by many people prominent in psychiatry who felt that the most important part of raising a child was to eliminate anxiety from his world. Neurotic parents, grasping this advice tenaciously, caused just what they so desperately wished to avoid. When the child is overprotected from the rigors and realities of the world he is not able to develop the ego strength needed to cope with existing conditions. As he grows older he becomes anxious because he cannot then be protected completely. Lacking the ego strength to handle anxiety-provoking situations, he soon begins to realize that anxiety must be avoided at all costs. Furthermore, his neurotic position is reinforced because the child reasons that anxiety must really be dangerous, for if this were not true, why should his parents protect him so diligently? Both his overprotected world, which results in weak ego function, and his excessive parental-induced fear of anxiety combine to lay the basis for neurosis.

Later in life, as he is required to face more realities, both internal and external, many of which are necessarily fraught with anxiety, he strives at all costs to avoid this reaction. In doing so, he develops a neurosis, because of his weakened ego. Whether it is a symptom neurosis, anxiety neurosis, or character neurosis depends on many factors in each case. Although the standard texts have delineated in detail many of the conflicts which take place in the neurotic relationship between parent and child, these texts have not stressed enough that such a relationship develops in a total setting where *anxiety is made so fearful and so dangerous* that the child is not able to develop effective ego defenses to handle his fear.

The second cause of neurosis, in which the parent is so filled with anxiety that he passes this burden on to his child, is probably less important in our society. Certainly this transference causes neuroses, but at least it is out in the open where the child can try to handle it. If he cannot, he may also develop inordinate fears and take the neurotic path, although children can cope with surprisingly large amounts of direct anxiety and anxiety-provoking situations. In fact, there is evidence to show that in the most difficult situations such as concentration camps and other severe environments, the children fared as well as or better than the adults. This is exemplified in many accounts and stories of actual happenings such as in Anne Frank's book, *The Diary of a Young Girl*[1] or a more recent book, Michel del Castillo's *Child of Our Time*.[2]

Children must be treated realistically and not insulated from the discomforts and the necessary rules of the world. If they cannot develop enough effective ego strength to handle discomfort and to obey the rules while they are under the

[1] Doubleday & Company, Inc., 1958; Random House (Modern Library ed., 1958).
[2] Alfred A. Knopf, Inc., 1958.

guidance of loving parents, when will they learn? They may learn under other circumstances, but they will have missed the best opportunity to develop this necessary ego strength. Instead of fearing and running from discomfort or from anxiety engendered by discomfort, the child must learn to use anxiety for its true purpose, which is a warning that the ego is not functioning as well as it might. The person with an effective ego, using anxiety as a stimulus to better ego functioning, may suffer in many cases, but if there is something which can be done, he tries to do it. Thus follows the basic psychological lesson: Hardship and anxiety are not to be feared and fled from but dealt with or tolerated until the situation changes. What better opportunity is there to learn this lesson than in relationship with non-fearing parents whom the child loves and trusts?

Following are two examples of situations in which neurosis is bred. In many middle-income homes every effort is made to spare the child the knowledge that money is a scarce and valuable commodity. Perhaps sacrificing themselves to this end, the parents often find that the result is opposite from what they had desired. When the child eventually finds out what the real situation is, he has no way to handle it psychologically or realistically. He may then hate his parents for perpetrating this unreality on him, or he may fail to function effectively and be a burden to them as long as they live. He may also take one of many neurotic pathways out of the situation, such as obsessively saving money, negligently spending it, or turning to alcohol. The situation is similar where parents, fearing that their child may be inhibited sexually as they might have been, do everything possible to allow free sexual expression. Again, this attitude provides difficulties for the child later on, when he finds that the world does not accept his behavior. In both of these situations, it is seen that the parental attitude, in which the parents fear to allow their child to fear, has laid the foundations for neurosis.

10

The Changing Manifestations of Neuroses

THE PICTURE OF NEUROTIC EGO FUNCTIONING IS CHANGING in our present society. The types of symptom neuroses which Freud saw in Vienna sixty years ago are rarely seen in a modern American psychiatric practice. Today the type of patient who comes for psychiatric help and who makes up a large part of all psychiatric practices might not have been recognized as mentally ill by the pioneers of psychiatry. This does not mean that the early discoveries are no longer applicable in understanding the neurotic of our time; it does mean, however, that we must be prepared to modify our thinking as the picture of neurosis continues to change.

The classical neuroses are the symptom neuroses which will be discussed in detail in the next chapter. Severe and psychologically crippling as some of them are, they do allow the basic ego structure to remain relatively intact in many people who suffer from them. As will be pointed out, such people suffer from a specific ego weakness which leads to the neurosis, although in other respects they often have a fairly effective functioning ego. Instead of erecting elaborate character defenses against their anxiety, they have settled for a neurotic symptom. Their difficulty is confined to one area, often, as Freud found out, that of inhibited expression of the need for sexual gratification.

Sexual inhibition was not uncommon in the more puritanical, Victorian era of the late nineteenth and early twentieth centuries. Fair maidens swooned at the mention of anything with a sexual connotation and, young blades thrilled at the rare sight of an exposed and shapely ankle. Furthermore, the family was a tighter unit than it is today, with the roles of the parents better defined. A strict father was head of the house, and the mother was a busy but more passive participant in the family activities. Sex was an activity which was not mentioned. In direct conflict with the biological needs, fear and anxiety regarding sex was present and symptom neuroses flourished.

This fear and anxiety, however, was counterbalanced by the tightly knit family situation where the roles of male and female were definite and where the children were taught the rules and regulations of society. Thus, in an atmosphere where much tended to produce strong egos, there was one subject, sex, which was laden with fear. The groundwork was laid to produce a specific ego weakness in what was otherwise a fairly strong ego. One of Freud's great contributions was psychoanalysis, in which the free expression of these sexual feelings often led to a dramatic cure of the symptom neurosis. This is the way it used to be, but times and neuroses have undergone drastic change.

The great social upheavals wrought by World War I marked the beginning of the end of the "good old-fashioned" symptom neuroses. Infrequently seen today, when present they are often a mask for underlying psychosis. The social changes produced a confusion in sexual roles as women became emancipated and took over more activities which were previously masculine prerogatives. Family structure loosened, divorce became more accepted, and the father lost his patriarchal position. The era of prohibition and its alcoholic and sexual concomitants further relaxed the Victorian and puritanical morality of the country. The fatalistic philosophies produced by the death, destruction, and destitution of World War I continued: to live for the present as suggested in *The Rubáiyát of Omar Khayyam* became more the vogue.

The twenties were followed by the social disintegration of the thirties when great industrial institutions vanished, banks closed, and poverty was rife. The whole nation, gripped by anxiety, elected a "radical" President and a Congress who, acting upon the need to alleviate the national anxiety, legislated measures which are the basis for much of our present political structure based on security. After the Depression came World War II and with it the completion of much of the loss of sexual identification and family structure initiated by World War I.

With these great social changes neuroses changed. Anxiety neuroses became more common as the ego became generally weaker during this era of the loosening of family ties and of less well-defined models for correct sexual identification. Character neuroses, based on the fear of anxiety, with the whole character involved in the effort to reduce anxiety, are growing in frequency. Immorality is much more tolerated, even encouraged, by a national attitude of personal laissez faire. No more classic example of this pattern is the hoodwinking of a whole nation uncovered in the television scandals of 1959 so loudly denounced, but quickly forgotten in our acceptance of wrong and our pious pseudopsychologically inspired pity-don't-censure attitudes toward the wrongdoers.

Homosexuality and the sexual neuroses are increasing because of the inability of many children to make a strong, positive sexual identification; this inability is, in turn, caused by the increasing breakdown of well-defined sexual roles. Ego weakness in our present society is more generalized, and increasing numbers of character neuroses are the result. Today the problem is not the specific ego weakness of the symptom neurosis but the generalized ego weakness of the character neurosis, which is much more difficult to treat.

11

Specific Ego Weakness— Neurotic Symptoms—Symptom Neuroses

THE SYMPTOM NEUROSES RESULT FROM A VERY SPECIFIC EGO weakness. In these cases, although a large part of the ego may be intact and functioning well, there are specific areas which are weak. As explained previously, neurosis is defined by the amount of ego weakness as well as by the method which the ego uses to handle anxiety. In symptom neuroses much of the ego is usually intact and strong. The areas of effective ego may, in fact, be strong enough so that except in the area of their neurosis people with symptom neuroses may function very effectively. It must be postulated that in their ego development they had enough good relationships with people with effective egos to account for the condition in which only a portion of their ego is weak.

In the following discussion, it is shown how the character defends pathologically against a specific weakness. In such cases the character tries to eliminate the anxiety inherent in the situation where there is an ego weakness. The method by which the character does this produces the symptom neurosis. The particular type of neurosis produced depends upon which of several methods the character uses. In all cases the character tries to eliminate the anxiety by substituting a neurotic symptom for the anxiety. The neurotic symptom (or symptoms, as there may be more than one) drastically reduces the ability of the ego to function properly in a certain area. The reduction in ego function is the price that the person pays for the partial elimination of the anxiety. The type of symptom neurosis is named by the neurotic symptom which predominates. Thus, to recapitulate, a symptom neurosis can be illustrated by the following circle:

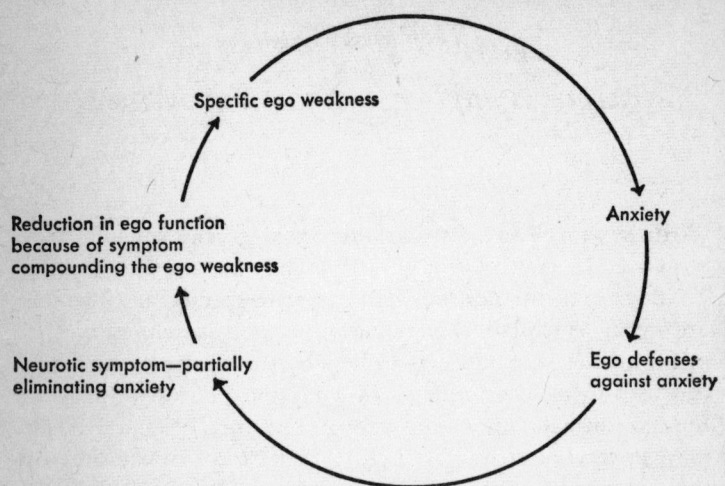

The process of the symptom neurosis, by producing a neurotic symptom, thus aggravates the initial ego weakness, and the process repeats in a circular fashion. As the ego weakness is intensified the neurotic symptom or symptoms become more pronounced to try to compensate for the greater anxiety produced by the increased ego weakness. The whole process, perpetuating and self-increasing, is similar to that of a person trying to escape a treadmill. As such a person may run until he falls from fatigue, so may a person with a neurosis that continues unchecked have a nervous breakdown. Fortunately the process is usually checked at a level which the neurotic person can maintain without breakdown. However, for all practical purposes he loses a large segment of ego, and, unless psychotherapy or something else fortuitous intervenes, this part of his ego is permanently lost. This is the ultimate price which he pays to reach a state of balance with his neurosis.

To illustrate, let us observe the man with a phobia, a common and typical symptom neurosis. Of the many types of phobias probably the most widely known is claustrophobia —fear of closed spaces and close, crowded quarters. The man with claustrophobia appears normal in all respects except that in closely crowded places he becomes extremely and unreasonably frightened, suffering intense anxiety. He will fight, run, push, and do anything to get out of the crowded situation. If forced to stay he may go into an acute panic state and faint, thus removing himself from the situation by loss of consciousness. Here is how this phobia follows the circular pattern of neurosis.

Specific Ego Weakness

The man first had a specific ego weakness, manifested by his ego's inability to function effectively in filling its general protective function while he was in a closely crowded situation.

Anxiety

In this situation he suffers from overwhelming anxiety because of the specific defect in his ego functioning.

Ego Defenses
(Elaborated To Reduce the Anxiety)

He builds up in his character a whole catalogue of defenses which become part of his pattern of ego functioning. He stays away from crowds or situations where close quarters might exist. He says that people annoy him, that he prefers the wide open spaces, that he enjoys solitude or just the company of a few friends. He hates movies or plays because they are crass and commercial; restaurants are treacherous places where one can get poisoned, and any crowded situation is no good. Denying reality, projecting, and rationalizing, he has a hundred reasons why only small, intimate groups are satisfactory. He may even sublimate by playing with tin soldiers, in an adult way of course, claiming his hobby is Civil War battles. Thus his whole character structure, his pattern of ego function and defenses, is molded to avoid being in a closely crowded situation.

Neurotic Symptoms

Along with these character defenses he develops a phobia of which he may not be conscious, although everyone else is fully aware that "poor old George" has claustrophobia and he really becomes "panicked" in a crowd. The phobia may extend to small groups and strange places. He may even become acutely uncomfortable watching a basketball game on television when the camera shows shots of the crowd.

Reduction in Ego Function

Because of the phobia he avoids all situations where there are crowds or close quarters. If, for example, he is a salesman, he is able to sell to his own customers, perhaps doing a brilliant job, but he can't go to the company conventions. He avoids, if possible, visits to the main office where large groups may congregate in small rooms. He can't be promoted to sales manager because he can't stand the atmosphere of the sales office. He is not able to call on bigger customers because he can't "wine and dine" them—large, crowded restaurants terrify him. Reconciled to the loss of a large part of normal functioning, he is limited in his range of actions because of his symptom neurosis—a type of claustrophobia. If he tries to push himself into crowded situations he suffers so much anxiety that all his functioning is impaired, compounding the whole problem. He settles for the phobia therefore, with the resultant limitation of ego function.

Thus we see a man whose character has been molded by his anxiety following an original specific ego weakness. Suffering a specific loss of function in one area, in other areas he is quite normal. This example illustrates the principles of a specific ego weakness and how it can produce the complicated pathological process known as symptom neurosis.

In the next part of the chapter the various types of symptom neuroses are briefly discussed. The symptom neuroses are identified by the symptoms prominent in each type. Although on occasion symptom neurosis may be mixed or variable, such cases are fairly uncommon because the symptom is related to the specific ego weakness which in turn is part of the fixed character structure. As character does not change easily, the type of symptom neurosis usually stays the same. Quantitative variation may occur—the neurosis may be mild or severe—but rarely is there variation from one type to another.

Symptom Neuroses

The symptom neuroses may be grouped into four major types. These are:

1. Hysteria or conversion reactions.
2. Hypochondriasis or hypochondriacal neurosis.
3. Phobias.
4. Obsessive compulsive neurosis.

Hysteria or Conversion Reactions

The person suffering from hysteria has a characteristic mechanism of neurosis in which the pathological defense mechanism of denial is prominent. Denial is used first to try to counteract the anxiety caused by the ego weakness, but this attempt fails. It is then used to block out a whole area of either physical or mental functioning, and at this time it succeeds. This anxiety, itself disappearing because it is *converted* into one of a large group of physical or mental defects, nevertheless leads to the neurosis. Typical examples of this kind of neurosis or conversion reaction are the whole gamut of physical infirmities known as hysterical blindness, deafness, paralysis, anesthesia or loss of feeling in body areas, types of sexual impotence, and types of sexual frigidity. Mental symptoms may be blackouts, lapses of memory, and full-fledged amnesia.

Whether the symptom is mental as in memory loss or physical as in hysterical blindness, the point to be understood is that function is always lost. Varying in severity and duration the symptoms wax and wane, with symptom-free periods in between. Also in hysteria, symptoms may change: for example, it is not uncommon for a "paralyzed" leg to change to a leg without feeling or vice versa. Another typical finding in hysteria is that the symptoms are not truly physiologic—they do not follow the same path that true organic defects would have to follow. Pointing out to an hysteric person who has no feeling in his hand and good sensation in his forearm that such a condition is impossible physiologically because of nerve distribution has no effect on the patient's symptom.

The French psychiatrists have coined a term for the attitude which hysterical people have toward their symptom. They term this attitude *la belle indifference,* beautiful indifference, an excellent characterization of the slight concern hysterics have for their handicap. Generally hysterical symptoms are found more among the unlearned and superstitious groups and among people of average and below average intelligence than among sophisticated, fairly intelligent people.

In conversion reaction or hysteria, the patient is remarkably free of anxiety—it intervenes when the neurotic symptom is given up. For example, a person with a severe tic or facial muscle spasm who is temporarily cured of his tic will usually substitute another, perhaps worse, spasm to take its place. The object of therapy is to help the patient strengthen the particular ego weakness responsible for the symptom. Because he must experience some anxiety to accomplish this, in his treatment he must learn to handle the anxiety. If he can do so, he can be permanently helped; if not, although his symptoms may change in degree and location, they will continue. For the patient the hysterical symptom always has a meaning, usually not difficult to ascertain. For example, the person suffering from hysterical blindness may take that course to defend himself against seeing things which arouse sexual feelings or of which he is frightened. The earliest and most complete psychological work has been done on this aspect of hysteria. These fascinating studies retain much of their validity today.

Hypochondriacal Neuroses

The hypochondriacal neuroses, which are very common, are reciprocal, in some respects, to the conversion hysterias. In the conversion reactions the neurotic anxiety disappears because it is converted into a symptom which actually incapacitates the patient, e.g., hysterical paralysis. In hypochondriasis, the person has imaginary illnesses but no real physical or mental incapacity. Hypochondriacal illnesses, are generally attached to major organs and simulate real organic illness such as heart disease, bowel and stomach disease, or cancer of various organs.

Patients with such illnesses demand treatment and care for a variety of mild psychophysiologic reactions as well as for many completely imaginary symptoms. They read the slick magazines and develop every disease discussed. Demanding reassurance from their doctor that they are really sick, they become incensed when he refuses to go along with their neurosis and run from one doctor to another in an endless search for sickness. As long as their symptoms are "treated" they exhibit amazingly little anxiety, almost reveling in their illness. When they are no longer able to convince anyone that they are sick, they become anxious and upset, and try desperately to persuade someone that they are seriously ill. Needing the love and attention which sickness can attract, they use this neurosis for getting it. Hypochondriasis is a neurosis not limited to human beings, for even some domestic animals exhibit this same behavior, acting sick under certain circumstances for attention.

Hypochondriasis should be distinguished from malingering. The hypochondriac sincerely believes that he is ill and stops work when he feels too sick; the malingerer feigns illness to avoid work. The price a person pays for a hypochondriacal neurosis is a severe and widespread loss of functioning because, imaginary or not, his illness is real to him.

Despite some similarities in this neurosis, when it is severe, to mild psychosomatic illness, for the most part the difference is distinct. In hypochondriasis there is no organic damage although due to psychophysiologic reactions there may be a mild loss of actual function. In psychosomatic illness, to be discussed in Chapter 17, there is real damage to one or more organs and a different ego defect is involved.

Phobias

Phobias are specific and irrational fears attached to a particular situation, place, or person. The mechanism of the phobia has been well described in the explanation of claustrophobia which introduced this chapter.

As in the hysterias, the meaning of phobias can often be determined after consultation with a patient. Although it is not uncommon for the patient himself to understand the reason for a phobia, the fear remains unchanged. Phobias are difficult to treat. As in all neuroses the phobic person must experience anxiety in his treatment and, for treatment to be successful, he must develop ways to handle the anxiety without the phobia. Phobias are much more resistant to change than are hysterical symptoms. For example, a man who is claustrophobic usually stays claustrophobic and does not give this up for another symptom. Phobias vary little in severity; in true phobia the person is absolutely terrified by the place, person, or situation which he fears. There are few degrees of terror, and if it is not real terror, it is not a phobia. A person who is frightened and uncomfortable while in an airplane may still be able to ride in one on occasion. This person has a fear, but certainly no phobia; for, while there are degrees of fear, there are rarely degrees of the terror characteristic of true phobic behavior.

Obsessive—Compulsive Neurosis

A person with this neurosis is "forced" to obey certain obsessions or compulsions or both. An example is the person who has the constant obsessive thought that he is going to drive his car into a crowd of people crossing on a crosswalk. This thought comes continuously and without surcease as long as the person drives his car in crowded places. He may have to give up driving where there is any degree of pedestrian traffic, or perhaps even give up driving altogether because of the thought and the fear of the consequences. If this neurosis were a phobia instead of an obsession the person would not be aware of the thought but would be afraid of all cars. In an obsessive neurosis the symptom is far different —the person may be comfortable driving in the suburbs or country and be perfectly at ease when someone else is driving. The obsessive thought, which in turn reduces function, is the basis of this neurosis.

Another common form which this neurosis takes is compulsive cleanliness and orderliness. The compulsive hand washer or house cleaner—the Craig's wife type of personality—becomes anxious unless everything is clean and in perfect order. In order to escape the anxiety he must go through certain self-dictated behavior—the compulsion. Usually fairly intelligent and often high up the socio-economic scale, he sometimes makes a good adjustment in large segments of the world because there are many jobs which require an obsessive attention to neatness and detail. In such a job, bank bookkeeping, for example, his neurosis may be an ally. In contrast to the phobias, obsessive–compulsive behavior and thoughts may vary considerably in degree. In strange or stressful situations the person may be so compulsive that he cannot function, whereas in quiet, familiar, safe situations he may function almost normally.

Usually in compulsive neurosis the whole character or personality is involved in the process. When we say he is compulsive, we mean he has a compulsive personality, which is, unfortunately, almost impossible to change. Often, however, the person finds a niche in life where he lives happily. Trouble starts when these people are put in positions of authority, which may occur because they do such a good job as subordinates. Here they fail miserably and drive everyone else "crazy" with their compulsiveness.

Industry, especially, has difficulty with this type of person, and he can also be disastrous in the armed forces. Such a personality was Captain Queeg in *Caine Mutiny* until, under severe stress, he became psychotic. By the time of the court-martial, however, he had returned partly to his old compulsive personality. In fact it was the defense lawyer's use of his knowledge of Queeg's personality which led to the court-martial's acquittal of the accused. This type of neurosis and personality borders very closely on psychosis. As in psychosis, the person is walling off a section of reality by bowing to the compulsion, and he is satisfying some needs within himself by his behavior. The difference is that in neurosis he is aware of what he is doing although he is powerless to change his behavior. Thus his need for achievement may be solved by an obsessive thought rather than in reality.

An example is the person who has the obsessive feeling that he is a success or a failure in whatever he is doing, although he may be far from it by actual standards. Although he realizes that his belief may be false, he cannot change it. Thus he differs from the psychotic who has no understanding of his unrealistic ideas. As was the case with all of the previously described symptom neuroses, the obsessions and the compulsions are used to avoid anxiety, and when they are thwarted the patient suffers. Also as before they have special meaning to the patient, although discovering this meaning is not the vital part of their therapy.

12

Generalized Ego Weakness— Anxiety Neurosis

IT HAS BEEN SAID THAT WE LIVE IN THE AGE OF ANXIETY. WE are searching for security, for adjustment, for freedom from tension. We constantly suffer from the gnawing fear that perhaps we are inadequate to deal with the complexities of our modern world. Many people long for the "good old days." That there is more than nostalgia in this yearning is shown by the fact that over one hundred million tranquilizer tablets of just one formula were consumed in the year 1957. For most of us, anxiety is something which we accept—a part of being alive today. Still, most of us do not have anxiety at all times, and we are able to control it by effective ego functioning.

There is, however, a large group of people in our society who are overwhelmed at all times by varying degrees of anxiety. Suffering from a generalized type of ego weakness, they are labeled anxiety neurotics. These people have an ego which is weak and frayed. Although it has no gaps or psychotic segments, it is far from the strong, flexible ego which produces effective ego functioning.

The person is filled with anxiety because his ego can neither fill his needs adequately nor protect him from the world. His ego is so weak that he has no fixed character structure with which to defend himself. He does not even use his poor defenses because he does not have the ego strength either to deny reality or to distort it to his advantage as do the character neurotics. Because he has enough ego to be afraid of the consequences, he is rarely hostile or aggressive. His ego, although weak and functioning poorly, is not shattered as are those of the people suffering from character disorders. Able to feel anxiety, he is not able to do anything about it. Besides being pathetic, easily panicked, nervous, and anxious, he suffers from all the physiologic symptoms of excessive anxiety and is thus afflicted both mentally and physically. One wonders with good reason what he gets out of life as he suffers almost continuously.

Although the anxiety neurotic is not uncommon, there is little helpful provision for him because he is not threatening to society. He is not feared as are the psychotic people, nor does he incur anger as do the severe character disorders. Scorned for his fear and weakness or pitied for his discomfort, little or nothing is done to help him. Perhaps completely unable to cope with the world, his ego may deteriorate to the extent that it is almost nonexistent. He may then be hospitalized and mistakenly labeled as a simple schizophrenic. If left alone his only hope is to gradually develop enough ego strength to get himself into a position where he suffers less and lives out his life in this manner.

Without sufficient ego strength to deal with his own impulses, he is terrified by ordinary feelings arising from his needs, for he knows that these needs must be satisfied in a world with which he can cope minimally at best. Because of his generally weakened ego he is caught between his needs and the world. He stands like a little man attempting to stop a fight between two enemy giants, of whom neither can seriously hurt the other although both are willing and capable of battering any third party in the way. He is the man in the way, taking a continual beating in the form of ever-present anxiety.

This type of person needs to have his ego strengthened—he has enough ego to suffer, but not enough to function effectively. He may benefit immensely from psychiatric help, although he does not have the type of ego abnormality which moves society to help him. Unfortunately he usually needs assistance from someone else to pay for his treatment because he is too anxiety-ridden to succeed in earning enough to pay by himself. There are the advantages, however, that he urgently desires help, and that while his ego and character are weak, they are not fixed. Psychotherapy can help him in many cases because, unlike a person with a character neurosis, he has not been able to develop pathological character defenses against anxiety. It is also interesting to note that from a psychiatric viewpoint the person who suffers from an anxiety neurosis is unusual because his psychiatric difficulty and his complaint are the same.

Intellectualizing-Rationalizing Anxiety Neurotic

This type of anxiety neurotic who suffers from overintellectualizing is not a textbook-recognized member of our neurotic society, but he should be. He talks too much and does little. Extremely common in our contemporary culture, he is moderately well accepted. The price he pay for his neurosis is literally talking himself out of accomplishing things in life. He overintellectualizes in an effort to avoid the consequences, emotional and physical, of really doing or feeling something. Worse off than the Walter Mitty person who at least lives in fantasy, he doesn't really live at all; he talks, argues, rationalizes, and gets uncomfortable around action.

He may be the intellectual "pink" who is all for the movement until it begins to move. Then he is terrified and quickly takes off in a new direction, often opposite from his original one. Knowing everything about everything, he does nothing about anything. Until he gets himself in a position where he has to put up or shut up, he is relatively harmless. Then, however, he becames immobilized, often with serious consequences to others if he has talked them into trusting him. His ego is similar to the ego of the anxiety neurotic except that he covers up his anxiety with talk. His ego reactions are all converted into intellectualization: he swoons at the sight of a powerful picture but runs from life. Universities give him a home as the perennial graduate student or perennial research assistant. Although he vehemently and vociferously opines on real life, he is a vocal rabbit. As society gets easier and further removed from the hard facts of reality, more and more he can find a place. In certain respected professions, such as our communications industry, he may be able to sell his neurosis for a good price because he can exist so insulated that he is never found out. These people, however, are parasites in any culture, and as they multiply the society suffers because their burden must be carried by someone else.

13

Generalized Ego Weakness— Character Neuroses

CHARACTER NEUROSIS IS THE MOST COMMON FORM OF ABnormal human functioning. As the social structure of our society becomes looser, character neuroses are increasing while symptom neuroses are decreasing. In distinction to the symptom neuroses, character neuroses often produce social problems because character neurotics often give vent to their feelings in antisocial ways. A character neurosis is basically, as are all neuroses, an ego weakness. It is not a specific ego weakness, but a general weakness in which a major portion of the ego is involved.

The symptom neurotic suffers because he uses his ego to try to compensate for his specific ego weakness, whereas the character neurotic uses the world to compensate for his more generalized ego weakness. Although the basis of a character neurosis is similar to the anxiety neurosis—both have fairly generalized ego weakness—there is almost no similarity in action.

Anxiety neurotics do not develop character neuroses because they have been raised in such a way that they learned to fear anxiety greatly. Character neurotics also have had initially a fear of anxiety, but, having been raised or put in a position where they have been able to learn to hate this fear of anxiety, they aggressively and actively do something to rid themselves of it. Whatever they do, they do with their whole characters. The result is the various types of character neuroses which are discussed in this chapter.

In character neurosis the whole personality takes over the function of ridding the weak ego of the hated–feared anxiety. When it is done successfully these people suffer little or no anxiety, but in order for this to occur others suffer because the character neurotics prey on others. When successful, they suffer less anxiety than any other group, for they experience anxiety only when they are prevented from fulfilling their needs in the world, which they attempt to do regardless of how they may hurt others. Unlike anxiety neurotics, who suffer internal anxiety, they suffer only from what can be described as external anxiety—that is, when they are prevented by the external situation from fulfilling their needs. This situation occurs because they are able to develop a character which functions only in accordance with what they perceive to be their needs.

Although they may recognize reality, they are interested only in what it can do for them. Only their needs are important, the needs of others have not the slightest meaning to them. They have decided that the way to avoid the anxiety engendered by their basically weak ego is to fulfill their needs and "to hell with everyone and everything" except themselves.

To explain this attitude in terms of ego function and character we must picture a group of people who have a one-sided ego. Their egos are concerned only with need satisfaction or with what their egos feel is need satisfaction. Anything in the world which does not pertain to their own need satisfaction they simply ignore, try to destroy, or alter so that it better fills their needs. They are often directly antisocial in their actions, as in the case of a person who writes bad checks, or indirectly, as in the case of the alcoholic who gets into trouble not from drinking but from drunkenness. Sooner or later they run into difficulty because providing unlimited need satisfaction is an arduous job for their weakened egos.

They find that even if they ignore everything besides themselves in the struggle for need satisfaction they are still unable to gratify themselves. They are thwarted in their attempt to go on their way ignoring everyone else—disregarding the rules of society without feeling any responsibility for their actions. In their frustrated search to fulfill all their needs and to use their egos to provide limitless pleasure they settle for a compromise. The compromise may be expressed by their use of an ego anesthetic such as alcohol, which they seize avidly. The alcohol blots out the anxiety and serves as a pleasant substitute for all that they cannot obtain from reality.

The alcoholic serves as a good example of the myriad of character neuroses because if the functioning of an alcoholic is understood, the mechanism of character neurosis becomes clear. An alcoholic is a person who derives all his satisfaction from the consumption of large quantities of alcohol. He lives to be drunk, because when he is drunk he feels pleasure in contrast to the pain of sobriety. An alcoholic will drink almost anything in the hope of getting drunk, although some have beverage preferences. Many alcoholics prefer to drink alone, because then there can be no interference with this pleasure activity. The alcoholic gets drunk because he wants peace and contentment from the anxiety which plagues him when he is sober. Thus we see a person with a basic generalized ego weakness who has decided that he must avert himself from the anxiety indigenous to this type of ego defect.

From ancient times alcohol has most commonly provided

the vehicle by which one can escape discomfort. Alcohol acts to reduce the anxiety and provides the illusion of fulfilling his needs. When anxiety derived from the drinking occurs, the alcoholic solves that problem by more drinking. His whole character settles for this satisfaction, thus defining a character neurosis. Unless he is able to strengthen his ego, he is doomed to alcoholism. Under pressure from a wife, relative, or friend, he may try to curb his drinking. Currently, an accepted way is to join Alcoholics Anonymous, an organization whose methods have been more successful than any others in helping alcoholics. In A.A., the alcoholic has two possible therapies. First, people who share his problem and whom he can accept are willing to try to help him satisfy his needs in a more socially acceptable way. Secondly, A.A. stresses ego strength through nondenominational religious faith. Even with the help of A.A., the problem is most difficult because he has found a way through alcohol to what he considers satisfaction. Although he occasionally seeks help through psychiatric treatment, he will rarely give up the bird in the hand for the promise of better birds in the bushes of psychiatry. In Part III there is further discussion of the therapy of alcoholics and character neurotics in general.

The remainder of this chapter is devoted to specific character neuroses. They are divided into two main groups, the oral or acting-in neuroses, and the acting-out neuroses.

The Acting-in Neuroses

Prime examples of people with acting-in neuroses are: alcoholics, pill or medicine takers, some types of tobacco users, marijuana and non-opiate drug users. The oral or acting-in neuroses are so named because the neurosis is expressed in the form of ingesting some substance such as alcohol or non-opiate drugs. This action, a compromise on the part of ego, provides these neurotics with the satisfaction they so desperately need. Although passive rather than basically antisocial, they often engage in antisocial activity. Without ability to delay satisfaction, paying a price that may include physical or mental breakdown, they ignore the end result and live for present pleasure. The alcoholic has been discussed in the previous section so that little need be added here. Few people can live a lifetime in the "civilized" world without having known at least one alcoholic. Alcoholism is as old as man, and probably even the cave man was acquainted with this balm to anxiety, the most ancient of all tranquilizers.

Using a different means of expression but suffering from the same problem are the pill takers, most of whom are habituated to the Benzedrine drugs, the barbiturate drugs, or mixtures of the two. There is a whole group of additional people who use other drugs such as marijuana, cocaine (as did Sherlock Holmes) and the mescaline, peyoti drugs. None of the latter, however, add up to anywhere near the problems or numbers of the alcoholics, probably because alcohol is both more socially acceptable and easily accessible. Marijuana usage is serious mainly because it may lead to heroin addiction. Heroin addicts are not character *neurotics* but are suffering from the more serious character *disorders*. They should be classed under character disorders because their ego is fragmented, in contrast to the very weak but still intact ego structure of the character neurotics.

Tobacco addiction may be classed as a character neurosis in the case of one definite disease, Buerger's disease, and probably in several less definite cases such as heart and lung disease. In these cases the need for inhaling tobacco smoke for satisfaction is so great that the person may do so at the risk of his life or limbs. Buerger's disease is characterized by a deficient blood supply to the arms and the legs and especially to the hands and feet. Although tobacco seems to act specifically in cutting down the little remaining blood flow, it is almost impossible to persuade these people to give up smoking. They may lose their hands and feet from dry gangrene due to deficient blood supply but they continue to smoke. Some people continue to smoke while suffering from certain heart or lung diseases, although here the relationship

GENERALIZED EGO WEAKNESS—CHARACTER NEUROSES

is not as clear-cut as in Buerger's disease. Other than in these cases, however, the users of tobacco cannot be described as character neurotics.

Finally, the food addict should be mentioned. Using food as others might use alcohol, he stuffs himself, becoming obese and unattractive, and then stuffs himself more as his unattractiveness makes life more difficult. The overeating often continues until excessive weight may endanger his life.

All these people derive temporary satisfaction from the neurotic pathway which they choose, the satisfaction coming through the portal of the mouth. They are all extremely resistant to psychiatric treatment, and much research is being done in an effort to improve the treatment which psychiatry can offer. As with the symptom neuroses, part of the basic treatment is to get them to accept some anxiety. How this may be done is discussed in Part III.

ACTING-OUT NEUROSES

The acting-out neuroses are in contrast to the acting-in neuroses discussed in the previous pages. In the acting-in neuroses the neurotic symptoms involved ingesting a substance which in turn becomes a substitute for effective ego functioning. In acting-out neuroses the whole character is devoted to some activity to obtain satisfaction and keep down the level of anxiety. In this process reality is ignored or denied, and other people are used and manipulated in a completely selfish manner.

The whole group of habitual gamblers, white-collar criminals, con men, swindlers, forgers, petty thieves, and gross thieves fit into this class. Also representative are the people who "never make the grade"—the black sheep or prodigal child who indulges repeatedly in a variety of activities leading to trouble. Amid tearful scenes wherein the prodigal swears reform, his parents bail him out of one difficulty after another in an endless process which leads in many cases to the disintegration of a family.

Devoid of conscience and without honor, these people use any form of activity to gain their ends. Having no feeling for anyone except themselves, they are at a loss to understand feelings in other people. They don't even understand how they hurt others in their activities because their egos are so completely oriented toward self-satisfaction. In their continuous activity they feel no real anxiety. Even when they engage in criminal activities, they feel excitement (not anxiety) to be pitting their wits against society. Having no regard for law and order they feel that honesty is for suckers. In an attempt to justify their activity they quote common rationalizations such as, "You can't cheat an honest man." Occasionally they may be successful in business because they are not bound by moral standards which their competitors obey, and because often they are witty, charming, and pleasant. They exude confidence, ease, and *savoir-faire* so that, while we often enjoy their company, we can be easily victimized if we do not recognize them for what they are.

If the activities of the acting-out neurotics are illegal, putting them in a correctional institution is only a mild restriction because they soon have the whole place "organized." In fact, often they do better while in jail than out of jail because some of their basic needs, such as food and shelter, are provided, leaving them free to manipulate the inmates and guards to their own advantage. Living by no law except their own, they fit anywhere as long as they are free to "operate."

This type of character neurotic is a person whose whole ego is dedicated to the proposition that anything is fair as long as it's for him. Intolerable anxiety may occur if he starts to obey the rules and regulations of society. Even in a position of high status where following the rules would be easy, he finds this course impossible. Examples are physicians who become abortionists or who sell narcotics that they may buy legally. Although the apparent gain is small compared to the possible loss, a few do it all the time. To them the accepted course is intolerable even if it is better by all standards of logic.

Character neurotics are extremely difficult to help psychiatrically. When they occasionally are seen by psychiatrists it is usually because all other paths are closed. Rarely motivated to change, they try instead to use the psychiatrist to help them continue on their way. Even if they cannot fool the psychiatrist, they try to use him indirectly when they are arrested and tried, by telling the judge that "anyone who acts like me must be crazy." They then sometimes get enforced psychiatric treatment, a "punishment" considerably better than a jail sentence. Because they have no understanding of their condition, the psychiatrist treating these people must initially work toward getting them to realize that they need long-term help.

This therapeutic task is so difficult that many psychiatrists, having been "burned" a few times by this type of patient, will not see them for therapy. Such a refusal gives the character neurotic even more ammunition, for he can then ridicule the psychiatrist as being helpless and worthless in his profession because he can't quickly solve all the neurotic's problems. The character neurotic conveniently ignores the fact that he does not want psychiatric help, only to get off the hook. If he is to be treated successfully, the psychiatric treatment has to be in a situation where the psychiatrist is in control; that is, he must be treated in institutions except under most unusual circumstances where someone can be hired to enforce socially acceptable behavior and prevent his usual activities.

The acting-out neurotics, as is evident, have such weak character structures that they can never form good relationships. It is tragic when they marry and have children, for they can give them nothing worthwhile. In fact, they often victimize their own children as soon as it is advantageous to do so. They may marry many times, often without benefit of divorce, justifying themselves with the delusion that they are God's gift to women or men. With no more conception of marital responsibility than any other kind, they often bring heartbreak to unsuspecting mates.

All the acting-out character neurotics are extremely undesirable members of society. They are far worse than the oral character neurotics because they prey on other people. Occupying a large part of our adult custodial facilities, they, together with the character disorders, comprise almost the total antisocial population. These two groups are increasing in numbers as our society becomes looser, with less stress on individual responsibility. They can cause the breakdown of any society if they get in control because all their activities are ultimately socially destructive.

14

Special Character Neuroses— Sexual Neuroses

THE SEXUAL NEUROSES, WHICH INCLUDE HOMOSEXUALITY and various forms of sexual perversions, are very specific kinds of character neuroses. The same basic mechanism—an ego weakness concerning sexual identification—underlies all of the sexual neuroses. People who suffer from sexual neuroses are confused because they are unable to accept their biological sex. An outgrowth of this confusion, the sexual neurosis, is an attempt to find a sexual identity, but it is a neurotic attempt because reality is ignored or distorted. The price the person pays for this attempt is abnormal sexual activity with a resultant lack of normal sexual satisfaction. Because of confusion about his sexual identity, the sexual neurotic forfeits the possibility of truly satisfying his strong basic sexual needs and accepts a compromise.

To understand almost all sexual neuroses it is necessary to appreciate the importance of correct sexual identity. As discussed early in this book, the person with an effective ego has a strong, positive sense of identity. He knows who he is sexually, that is, male or female, and he knows who he is relative to other people in the world. People with sexual neuroses do not know who they are sexually. They are not sure of their sexual role, but they are searching for the solution to their problem. A mature man with an effective ego accepts the normal function of his sexual organ. He also accepts the fact that women do not have an external sexual organ but have the female receptive genitalia. Similarly a mature woman accepts her sexual role: she accepts the fact that she does not have an external sexual organ but does have internal organs. Under proper circumstances she readily accepts pregnancy and childbirth.

Although the acceptance of the natural sexual role may seem simple as described here, it is not at all simple for many people in our society. Unsure of just what sex they are, these people, of both sexes, are far from convinced that their sexual anatomy is either proper or adequate for their sexual role. Although the confusion over sexual identity is largely a psychological problem, the method which the sexual neurotic uses to solve his problem centers itself in the concrete physiological denominator of sex, the sexual organ. The male who is unsure of his sex is convinced that his sexual organ is not capable of playing the proper male role. Dominated by the feeling that he is sexually different from other males, he feels an emptiness, an unsureness, and a growing anxiety due to this basic sexual confusion. He knows he is not a woman, but does not feel like a man. This leaves him in the middle, for there are only two teams in this game and he feels he is not a member of either one. Similarly, a woman refuses to accept the fact that she has so little anatomically to show for her sexual role. Feeling cheated, she will not accept the fact that males have been so much more generously endowed with sexual anatomy. She can't bring herself to accept the passive role of a woman because that would be admitting that she will never have anything more than she has now. Try as she may, however, there is no possible hope that sexually she will ever be a male, with all its concomitants of actively striving sexuality.

This middle position is the situation in which the sexual neurotic exists. He lives in the confused, poorly identified area between what is really male and what is really female. The particular sexual neurosis is his attempt to solve the problem and rid himself of the emptiness and anxiety inherent in the confusion of sexual identity. He may, as do many neurotics, function well in activities not directly related to his neurosis, although to do so he must develop elaborate defenses against his ego weakness in the area of sexual identity. In the homosexual the whole basis of his defense is love for people of the same sex. The feeling of love and attraction covers up his real feeling of sexual inadequacy. The homosexual is conscious only of the feeling of love for those of his own sex in contrast to the fear and anxiety he feels when he is cast into a heterosexual role. He is not conscious of what drives him to this compromise.

When the ego is weak in other areas in addition to sexual identity, a man may not develop homosexuality as a defense. He may act impulsively in dangerous, antisocial ways because of his inability to defend himself against the anger and frustration built up by the sexual ego weakness. He may take a myriad of other courses, ranging from a harmless Peeping Tom at one end of the scale to a dangerous homicidal sexual psychopath at the other end. Between the elaborate character defense for a homosexual and the poorly defended, poorly controlled sexual criminal, there is a vast gap. It is not psychologically sound to accept the present legal viewpoint which lumps all of these people together as sodomists. Although they have the same basic problems, we should be concerned as much with the type and stability of the actual neurotic expression as with the identity problem underlying their behavior. Whatever the expression, however, these people are suffering from a specific type of character neurosis. They deserve psychiatric care, not punishment.

Homosexuality—Male

In my opinion homosexuality in males is one of the most serious problems in our society. Homosexual men are increasing in greater numbers than women which eliminates supply of mates as a factor in male homosexuality, since there is a surplus of unmarried women in our society. Of course increasing numbers of homosexuals are contributing to this surplus. Our methods of helping these people are extremely poor. Our legal structure, which makes this neurosis a crime, is archaic, for there is no more reason to make this ego weakness a crime than to make a phobia a crime. The fact that some of the more severe sexual neuroses are dangerous does not mean all sexual neuroses, particularly homosexuality, are dangerous. This does not imply that homosexuality should be merely tolerated, but rather, that the concern of society about homosexuals should extend to making it possible and even attractive for them to seek help for their condition.

Ego Mechanism of Male Homosexuality

As explained previously, the male homosexual suffers from a sexual neurosis due to confusion about his sexual identity. Although his basic problem is psychological, it is manifested in a deep and undying concern that his sexual organ is not adequate. To escape from the anxiety inherent to this situation he has two choices: (1) he can try to take steps to reassure himself of the adequacy of his penis (the masculine homosexual role) or, (2) he can give up and accept the false premise that he is permanently inadequate (passive feminine homosexual role). In either case he will be homosexual. His decision affects only the form in which he expresses his homosexuality, whether he takes the masculine role or the feminine role. It is not uncommon for homosexuals to try both roles and occasionally to shift roles. This change is possible because the basic ego weakness is the same in each case.

The male homosexual is searching for a sexual organ which he feels is adequate, or for reassurance that his own is adequate. In the process his whole character changes to aid him in his search. He can try to become masculine enough to attract a feminine man who will become enamored of him, thus helping to reassure him that he must be all right because he has succeeded in attracting a passive feminine man; or he may take the feminine role in which he looks for a "stronger man" who can be enticed into a homosexual love affair or relationship. If he can accomplish the latter he has the feeling that the bigger, stronger organ is partly his. In neither case are sexual relations with a woman feasible because she has no visible sex organ. This absence frightens all homosexual men because they are reminded that, sexually insecure as they are, things could be even worse. They could, like women, have no external sex organ at all. On the other hand, the passive feminine male homosexuals are attracted to the company of women as long as there is no sex in the relationship. Realizing that women have the power to attract masculine men, they hope that by associating socially with attractive, feminine women they may acquire some of this power. They have the comforting feeling that they are all "girls" together.

It must be understood that, although homosexuals constantly discuss and stress how important large sex organs are, the actual size means very little, for their fear of sexual inadequacy is based on an unconscious ego weakness, not on their real anatomy. Thus, the homosexual male in some cases develops a supermasculine character, builds muscles and engages in "male" activities in an effort to reassure himself of his masculinity, as did the husband in the play *Tea and Sympathy*. More often, he takes the feminine role.

Assuming feminine characteristics of passivity to try to attract a masculine man, he may in extreme cases resort to surgery to remove his own sex organ in the hope that now, as a surgically created woman, he can finally get what he so desires—a strong man for himself. In any case his attempt fails because a normal masculine man will not respond.

No matter which role the homosexual chooses he must try to attract either a "masculine" or "feminine" homosexual, depending on his type. He may enter into a marriage arrangement with a woman so that he has a respectable front for his homosexual activities. Often he enters into a pseudo-marriage with a man or a long series of homosexual arrangements. By these means he resolves his problem neurotically and joins the homosexual society. Here he lives in the "gay" world surrounded and reassured by the many people who are like him and who can give him love and affection. When he casts his role with the "third sex" he has accepted his lot. Like a small boy at a peep show, he still gets a sly thrill out of talking about heterosexual relationships.

Accepting sexual inadequacy, he often tries to compensate for his lack of sexual identity by becoming arty, witty, and creative. He chooses this avenue for several reasons. If he achieves something in the fields where these characteristics are important, he gains a new feeling of identity which partially alleviates his emptiness. Also, these fields give him a chance to express indirectly his thwarted sexual feelings: he finds in painting, the theater, and music safe avenues for sexual feelings which he cannot express directly because he does not have sufficient identity. Finally, though by no means least important, there is the lack of a direct expression of masculinity in these pursuits. In the arts where there is so much sexual subtlety, there are so many nuances, he gains satisfaction by "playing" at sex tangentially. Here, where he feels comfortable, he may be active and striving, though it is never a truly masculine type of aggressiveness. For these reasons male homosexuals always make up a small but ever-present minority among the creative and artistically expressive people in any community.

Because the homosexual is not able to accept his sexual identity, he cannot really satisfy his need for sexual gratification. His frustration causes anxiety which is always close to the surface because he can never completely accept a situation—his homosexual role—in which a basic need remains unsatisfied. He is always engaged in a restless, continually frustrated search for a more satisfactory identity than the one he has settled for. This searching, "'cruising" as he calls it, often leads him into the hands of police decoys, who accept his homosexual advances and then arrest this unfortunate neurotic.

Although psychiatry at present can offer no completely successful way to remedy the homosexual's problem, it certainly seems unjust that this group is singled out for punishment by making their neurotic compromise a crime.

Homosexuality—Female

The female homosexual is not able to accept her identity as a woman. The basic mechanism is similar to that of male homosexuality. The female who, rationalizing because of her anatomy, feels cheated in her sexual role becomes an active "masculine" homosexual. Her problem stems from the fact that she does not have a male organ, yet she feels active sexual drives. She is unable to accept the thought of passive, receptive femininity. Although she cannot accept the male as superior, she fears the male sexual organ because it reinforces her lack of female identity by reminding her of what she will never have.

The female who plays the passive feminine role in the homosexual situation feels inadequate as a female rather than cheated. She accepts the love of the masculine woman because she feels unable to cope with the heterosexual responsibilities of a woman. By accepting homosexuality she gets more attention with less responsibility. In a sense she has no sexual identity, just a childish longing for love and protection. This type of woman has no counterpart in numbers among males although some very passive male homosexuals play approximately the same role. Such a woman, who has a much weaker character than the masculine female homosexual, has little identity in contrast to the usually strong identity (except sexually) of the "masculine" female homosexual.

Consciously the female homosexual desires the love of a woman because she feels that this is the only true, pure love, in contrast to heterosexual love which is dirty and degrading. She uses these two words often because they mean just what she feels: It is dirty because it implies ejaculation, and it is degrading because she is placed in the passive, subordinate position. This can't happen to an aggressive female homosexual when she loves a woman. With a woman who loves her she, at least, gets the psychological feeling that she has some degree of the masculinity for which she is searching. It would seem that loving a woman might upset a masculine female homosexual as it does the male. This does not happen because with a male she loses her whole fantasy by the objective sight of the penis she doesn't have while with a woman she can maintain the illusion.

Actually, however, female homosexuality is less prevalent and less serious because it is easier for a woman to acquire and accept her basic sexual identity. Almost all children have mothers with whom to identify, while in most cases fathers are less close so that there is less possibility for the formation of a good relationship. Also women have fewer sexual identity problems because their passive sexual role is easier to play than the active, striving male. Furthermore, it is easier to accept what was never there (a male sex organ) than it is to settle for what is there but at the same time is felt to be inadequate, as in the case of the male.

Because women homosexuals are almost never involved in aggressive sexual acts and because they make a far less obvious show of their homosexuality than do men, they are rarely involved with the law because of their behavior. Society tolerates women who live together far better than men who do the same thing, for society fears abnormal sexuality in males much more than in females. Finally, men as a group are probably more sexually insecure than are women;

thus the knowledge and sight of men who are homosexual is more threatening to males in our society. Since laws for the most part are made and enforced by men, it follows that our sodomy laws are more punitive toward male transgressors.

Latent Homosexuality

There is no doubt that almost everyone has some homosexual component in his character. Although none of us is completely secure in our sexual identification, this in no way implies that it is abnormal to have warm feelings and love for members of the same sex. There is a vast difference between homosexuality and the satisfactions afforded by the affection of a good friend of the same sex. Observers sometimes confuse these two relationships and read homosexuality into a situation when it does not exist, often causing much misery thereby. Apart from friendships, there are people who really do have some sexual confusion which may cause them to express a degree of homosexual behavior some time in their life. This again does not necessarily mean they are homosexual, because sexual identity develops with growth, maturity, love, and sexual relations. Few people arrive at their true level of mature sexual identity until well past adolescence. Finally there are people with a homosexual problem who never express it in actual homosexual behavior. Although it is probably correct to call them latent homosexuals, it is far more important to realize that they are successfully resisting this solution and that they need help toward developing more effective egos. Latent homosexuals should be protected from finding out that homosexuality is a part of their problem, for if they find out before they have enough ego strength to cope with these feelings, they can be made considerably worse.

Sexual Neuroses Other than Homosexuality

There are many sexual neuroses other than homosexuality. In each instance the mechanism is ego weakness concerning sexual identity; it is only the expression of this ego defect

SPECIAL CHARACTER NEUROSES—SEXUAL NEUROSES

which is different. Most numerous are the men who are afraid of women and women who are afraid of men. Both fear the opposite sex because of their own insecure, confused feelings about their sexual role. Afraid to be found out, they avoid the anxiety intrinsic to facing their confused sexual identity by avoiding the other sex. Society shows no concern with them because they merely abstain from sex. Living without mature sexual love, they sometimes compromise by showing affection for children, or animals, or even inanimate things such as pretty flowers.

The converse of this type is the satyr or nymphomaniac. These are the names for males (satyrs) and females (nymphomaniacs) who are sexually insatiable and whose whole life and character are directed to sexual conquests and activities. Don Juan is a literary example of a satyr, and recently a group of popular sex novels have been written about nymphomaniacs, prominent among whom was the heroine of *Forever Amber*. Again the mechanism is the same. In this case, because of a feeling of lack of sexual identity, the person indulges in excessive sexual activity to try to prove he or she is 100 per cent man or woman.

Although all of the previously discussed conditions fall into the group of sexual neuroses, they are differentiated legally and morally if not psychologically from the large group commonly called sexual perversions. Excluding homosexuality, which has been discussed in detail, the sexual perversions cover a wide variety of abnormal sexual activities. They range from relatively harmless members of this group to the dangerous sex sadist, a person legitimately feared in any society.

Almost all of the sexual perverts are men. Women occasionally masquerade as men, but they rarely engage in the other perverse types of sexual behavior. This is partly because they have a lesser problem with sexual identity and partly because women may behave in ways forbidden to men. For example, women may either expose themselves sexually in many blatant ways or dress in masculine clothes; men who attempt similar courses are immediately suspect. Finally, women are not basically sexually aggressive, so that their efforts to establish their identity would take a more passive course than do those of men who must be active to establish their true identity.

Because males are more active, male deviates are, in some cases, dangerous. Peeping Toms, fearful that they will not be accepted as males, restrict themselves to obtaining gratification by peeping and masturbating. Although they may be married, they still suffer from a gnawing sexual inadequacy which they solve in this manner. This activity, however, is much more dangerous to the peeper than to anyone else, for these people lay themselves open to aggressive retaliation when caught. Slightly more aggressive is the man who steals women's clothes. Despite consummating an act, he settles for a woman's belongings rather than for the woman herself. Next on the scale is the person who exposes himself sexually. He wants to be accepted as a man by means of public reassurance that he has a penis. He receives this reassurance, but he is usually locked up in the process. Although homosexuals occasionally dress as women, there is another group who masquerade without engaging in homosexuality. This activity is in direct opposition to the man who exposes himself. When a man masquerades as a woman in public he is sometimes jailed, although less often than the man who exposes himself. The difference is probably due to the more passive feminine action of the former.

There is the one group of sexually abnormal people who express their insecurity in an aggressive fashion. These are the people who attack young boys or girls, or even grown men and women. Again these attacks are their way to feel sexually powerful, to attempt to gain a sexual identity by aggressive sexual behavior. They may kill before or during the sexual attack, or even molest a lifeless body to gain omnipotence. They kill out of fear, powerless to stop the sexually aggressive activity which leads them to murder their victim to keep him from revealing their identity. They also kill because they feel sexually omnipotent when they destroy someone whom they feel is sexually inferior to them. They are unable to stop this perverse form of compensating for their sexual confusion. Thus these people are very dangerous. When they are discovered, they should be locked up for the purpose of treatment and not released until treatment is successful, even if this means lifelong institutionalization. These people are almost never homosexuals; if they were, they would not take this form of activity. Homosexuals, who take a nonaggressive, non-antisocial method of "solving" their problems, should not be confused with the aggressive sexual neurotics.

In all of these cases a responsible society owes sexual neurotics treatment, not punishment. The treatments are now long, difficult, and, unfortunately, often unsuccessful. Much research is needed to find more effective methods of therapy.

15
❖
Ego Thickness, Rigidity, Impenetrability— Psychosis

AT SOME TIME DURING HIS LIFE ONE OUT OF EVERY FOURteen people in the United States will be hospitalized for mental illness, according to recent statistics of the United States Public Health Service. Approximately half the hospital beds in this country are occupied by people suffering from a psychosis or a mental illness of such severity that hospitalization is required. The state of California alone spends over $121,000,000 a year just to take care of the mentally ill, most of whom are psychotic. This sum is required despite the fact that, in terms of ratio of mentally ill to total population, California is a relatively healthy state.

In popular or slang terms, a psychotic person can be described as crazy. In many respects crazy is a better word than psychotic or schizophrenic because it is better understood, and often elicits less fear than the more poorly understood terms of schizophrenia or psychosis. If it is said that Charlie has a crazy old aunt who lives with him, we are usually tolerant, but if the story is spread that Charlie has a schizophrenic or psychotic aunt, our reaction is apt to be more confused.

A psychotic person is chiefly distinguished by the way in which he deals with reality. Psychosis can be defined as a break with reality: the psychotic person does not act in the world realistically or as we would expect him to act. His behavior is bizarre, unpredictable, unrealistic. In his break with reality he may be described as out of contact; that is, he no longer responds to our attemps to communicate with him. In many psychotic people the most blatant evidence of this break is the observation that he experiences sensations which have no basis in reality. For example, he falsely perceives stimuli originating not in the world but within himself. These false perceptions are called hallucinations. Although hallucinations may occur in any of the senses, the most common by far are auditory. Hearing voices or sounds which are imaginary, the person may act according to commands of the imaginary voices. He is often the victim of false ideas called delusions, which may encompass anything from the idea that he is Jesus Christ to a simple thought that it is raining outside when the weather is clear. The point to be derived from this preliminary discussion is that it is possible for the psychotic person to behave in any way whatsoever, because his behavior may bear no relationship to the world around him.

To be psychotic, or crazy, one needs a certain type of ego structure. When this type of structure is understood, craziness makes sense because it is apparent that psychosis is the only available course. The ego of the psychotic person is complete and unbroken, but unlike the resilient, flexible, effective ego, it is rigid and thick-walled. This rigid ego fulfills the first condition of psychosis by serving as a wall or barrier between the person and the world. The ego is shown in the diagram as a thick, rigid wall closely surrounding the person. In the completely psychotic person this thickened ego completely surrounds the person. Rarely does this occur, so that most psychotics have an ego which is only partly thickened, part remaining relatively flexible and in contact with the world.

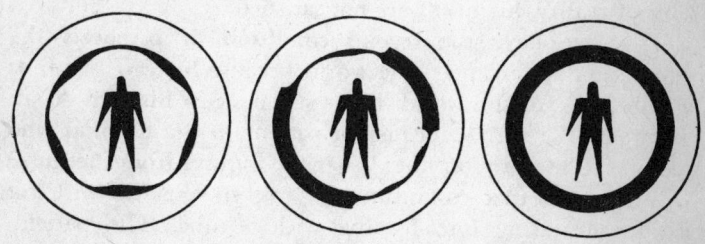

NORMAL   PARTIALLY PSYCHOTIC   COMPLETELY PSYCHOTIC

Keeping the functions of the ego in mind, it can be easily seen how this kind of ego produces highly abnormal behavior. The effective ego serves as a flexible connector between the person and the world, facilitating two-way contact, and mediating between the person's needs and the stresses of the world. In psychotic ego functioning this whole normal process is interrupted. Here the stresses of the world never psychologically affect the person, for the thick ego serves to separate him from the world. A psychotic patient in a mental ward may spend hours burning himself with cigarettes, feeling no pain, bemused at the smell of burning flesh. It is well known that at one time he had the capability of experiencing pain, but during the course of his severe psychosis, his thickened ego has walled off parts of the world. Thus he has lost the ability to feel certain external stimuli. This extreme example illustrates the first condition of psychosis by showing the amount of detachment which can be caused by a thick, rigid ego.

In the other direction the ego acts as a barrier between the needs of the person and their fulfillment in the world. A completely psychotic person is not able to fill any of his needs in the world because of the wall thrown up by his ego. This does not mean, however, that his needs go unfulfilled—it means that they go unfulfilled *in the world*. Actually they are partially or completely fulfilled within the thick-walled confines of his own ego. We call this method of satisfying needs "crazy" because, according to reality, or our conception of reality, his needs are not satisfied.

Thus we have the second condition of psychosis—the psychotic does not need the world because his ego stands as a substitute for the world. He is sufficient in himself. As an example: We may see a mental patient in the hospital who looks as if he were starving. When we inquire from the nurse why he is in that condition, she answers that he will not eat, necessitating force-feeding with a tube. The patient, however, may resist the tube feeding, complaining that he is not hungry and perhaps even stating that he has been eating satisfactorily. He has no perception of the realistic situation, only perceiving what his ego dictates. Without forceful intervention he may starve to death. Although this is a gross example, it well illustrates the second condition of psychosis.

Another patient may work out pages of complicated mathematical formulas dealing with a perpetual motion machine in order to satisfy part of his basic need for achievement. That these formulae have no basis in reality means nothing to him; in "his" reality, which is his own thick-walled ego, they are meaningful and satisfactory. In the joke described by William Saroyan when discussing an uncle who played only one note continuously on his bass fiddle, the uncle stated that he had found the note that all others were looking for. This illustrates the position of the psychotic patient, who has found in his ego a new and safer world. That this position is unrealistic is of no concern to him, because in-

EGO THICKNESS, RIGIDITY, IMPENETRABILITY

herent in his psychosis are two conditions: (1) the walling off of true reality, and (2) the substitution of a personal reality system for filling his needs completely within his own ego.

In psychosis the degrees of ego thickness may vary considerably. Although people who are totally psychotic do exist, they are rare. Totally psychotic, as mentioned previously, refers to a person whose ego is so thick-walled and closely bound around him that there is no contact at all between himself and the world. He may exist in this condition in a state hospital for years. In my personal experience I have known of a totally psychotic woman, huddled for forty-seven years, tube-fed and needing total care, in a "back ward" of a large state mental hospital. Such is the powerful barrier that a psychotic ego may throw up in the face of reality.

Although there may be large areas of the ego that are thick and rigid, as in most hospitalized, mentally ill patients, more often only a small section is rigid, as in the person who is only a little *eccentric,* a kind, euphemistic word which means slightly out of touch with reality. This type of person is exemplified by the neighbors who for years quarrel over the location of their property boundary, spending money for court actions and building huge fences out of all proportion to their disagreement. They have good contact and function well except in this one area, but here they are crazy in every sense of the word. Each has the delusion that the other is trying to harm him through this argument over their property. In this small area they act as if reality did not exist, which is the first step toward psychosis. The process may stop here or it may get worse. They may go on to believe that the neighbor is poisoning the ground in the garden, seducing their wives, or hexing their children. At this time they may get belligerent and threatening, so that they must be committed to a mental hospital.

Thus again we see the two conditions of a typical psychosis: (1) the ego first acts to wall off a small segment of reality, and (2) the person, for unique and personal reasons, then acts to fill some needs within this area of his ego. As this process waxes and wanes we see either full-blown psychotic behavior or a return to non-psychotic functioning. Unless a person is extremely aberrant in his behavior, or is actually threatening, we are fairly tolerant of his psychosis. Understanding that he has mental illness, we say, "Old Sam Jones is crazy as a coot, but he's harmless," and perhaps humor him or avoid him.

Psychotic ego functioning may vary widely. For example, when stress is increased a psychotic person is often able to act normally. This is illustrated by a person who seems psychotic until he is taken for commitment, when the sudden, added stress of being removed from home and locked up makes contact with his ego almost in the same way that a loud shot may be heard by a person who is hard of hearing. He then is able to mediate this extreme stress realistically. Acting rationally in the admission ward, he puzzles his whole family by resuming his crazy behavior shortly after he returns home. In other cases, however, increased stress turns a person away from reality toward psychosis because this added burden is more than his ego can effectively handle.

There are also people who seem to be able to turn psychosis off and on, acting crazy in certain situations, sane in others. An example in my experience was that of a husband and wife who were both psychotic when home together but who were rational in the hospital. If either the husband or wife was kept in the hospital while the other stayed home, both remained rational. The ward psychiatrist decided that the fairest course was to keep one in the hospital and one at home. After a period of time the one in the hospital would be discharged and sent home. In a short time both would become psychotic and the other would be brought back to the hospital, thus more or less equally dividing hospital time between husband and wife. Although admittedly this is an unusual case, it serves to illustrate vividly the changing character of psychosis.

Psychosis is a variation of ego functioning which is no

easy to understand even if the concept of a thickened, rigid ego is accepted. Although it is difficult to advance a theory which can explain how this type of ego develops, it can be postulated that psychosis begins with a susceptibility early in life. For reasons not fully understood by psychiatrists, the onset of psychosis may occur at any age. There are babies who seem psychotic almost from birth and, at the other extreme, an octogenarian may develop a senile psychosis after eighty years of effective ego functioning. These examples, however, are exceptions compared to the majority of patients who become psychotic during late adolescence through age forty.

In older literature psychosis was called dementia praecox, which meant precocious dementia or early mental illness. These cases began in the late teens, usually running a hopeless course with the victims, who received little or no treatment, dying in insane asylums. The age of onset of most psychoses has remained relatively unchanged, but the possibility of a cure due to better methods of treatment is now much greater.

Mention of the age of onset brings up the question of why psychosis occurs at *any* age? What happens to a person who "seemed" all right for many years that causes the ego to change at a later age to gross psychotic functioning? If one examines in detail the histories of psychotic patients, one fact stands out: they *didn't* get along all right, they just seemed to. The major defect is in the way they relate to other people, both within and outside of the immediate family. Consistently, from early in their lives, they are inherently unable to form a close, warm, loving relationship. They are distant, often to the point of isolation, seeming, in many cases, not to need more than the barest amount of human companionship. Parents often describe such children as good (in contradistinction to the other children), self-sufficient, and capable, preferring solitary amusements to associating with groups. Although this description does not imply that all such children are psychotic or destined to become psychotic, these tendencies are often the early pattern of people who later develop psychosis. If there is one phrase that psychiatrists hear from the mothers of psychotics, it is, "He was so good and didn't seem to need the love and attention that most children need." Before the break such persons usually are able to make the necessary relationships to some degree but they have to strain themselves to do so. In a crude attempt to remedy their inability to tolerate closeness, they are often forced by well-meaning family or friends into relationships of an intensity that they cannot handle. Although living in fear of closeness, they are not yet psychotic. In later years, under some stress, something goes wrong which leads to the ultimate ego thickening that is psychosis.

Although we can only postulate what goes wrong, fear which they feel when anyone gets too close is at the core of the problem. They fear because they were unable to respond emotionally in their early relationships. This inability to respond emotionally is often accentuated by mothers who are greatly dependent for their own gratification on these children. Because the children cannot relate with anywhere near the amount of emotional intensity that they sense is required, they fear retaliation by others, retaliation for what they unconsciously recognize as their inability to give closeness to a relationship. To avoid the fantasied retaliation they withdraw from other people. They become preoccupied with their own inner world, trying to find gratification of needs in fantasy rather than in reality. Finding the closeness they need within their own egos, they begin to depend more and more on this solution to their problem. As they grow more independent and isolated, others leave them more alone or try too late to get them involved in a relationship they can tolerate.

It is at this time that they need someone desperately, but they have lost the ability to make contact. They are now so isolated that only with great effort can they live in reality. As this process continues, they gradually or rapidly lose the incentive to make the effort. The degree of withdrawal varie greatly—some live more or less introspective, solitary lives, while others become blatantly psychotic.

The severity of the symptoms that these people exhibit is proportional to the amount of ego involved in the psychotic process as well as to the thickness of the psychotic ego. The content of the psychosis depends on the method which the thickened ego uses to fill the needs. No two psychotic people are alike, though they may outwardly exhibit similar symptoms and characteristics. These symptoms, whose meaning and content are beyond the scope of this book, are of some importance as they may aid a therapist to understand the illness. There is a large gap, however, between understanding the illness and helping the patient. Regardless of the therapy, it is important to understand that people are psychotic because of the thick, rigid ego which separates them from the world and acts as a substitute for reality.

16
❖

Psychosis—Specific Factors

Organic Psychosis

INITIALLY IT IS IMPORTANT TO DIFFERENTIATE BETWEEN ORganic and functional psychoses. The organic psychoses are those caused by a definite, known organic factor, whereas the functional psychoses are caused by factors of unkown origin. In this book the assumption is made that functional psychoses are psychological in origin, as described in the previous chapter.

Because no organic cause is found for the vast majority of psychoses, many psychiatrists subscribe to the belief that they are psychologically caused. At the present time, the receiving wards of mental hospitals admit very few psychoses of definite organic cause each year, while during the same time they admit many functional psychoses. Thirty to fifty years ago there were many patients in mental hospitals suffering from general paresis, the consequence of untreated syphilis. With the advent of penicillin this disease has been so controlled that only occasionally is a paretic admitted. Another large source of organic psychoses has been bromide, alcoholic and other toxic psychoses, but better medical treatment, together with physician alertness, has reduced the number of psychoses of these types. Excessive use of drugs such as cortisone or adrenal cortical agents can cause psychotic behavior. The most important organic psychosis today is senile psychosis, caused by changes in the brain due to aging. The number of people with this disease is increasing as medical science continues to make progress in lengthening the life span. When our culture was simpler we assumed more family responsibility in taking care of the old folks who developed senile psychosis; now there are large mental hospitals which every year assume the care of increasing numbers of elderly psychotics.

Whatever the cause, however, the actual ego defect in organic psychosis is similar to that in functional psychoses. The person with an organic psychosis loses part of the brain capacity needed to deal with reality in an effective way. He then takes what little ego function he has left, pulls it closely around him and uses it in place of reality. Many organic psychoses are manifestly impossible to tell from functional psychoses. Although unusual, it has happened that a toxic psychotic due to bromide poisoning is admitted to the hospital as a functional psychotic. It is possible that in hospitals where there is only one inexperienced doctor for five hundred patients the patient may be kept long after the bromide intoxication and its resultant psychosis have worn off. The more he protests his incarceration to untrained aides, the less he is believed. To avoid this particularly unpleasant situation many hospitals routinely check new patients for bromide poisoning.

Finally, the point should be made that not all people who are exposed to the same organic stress become psychotic. This implies, and I believe strongly, that even in many organic psychoses there is a large psychological element. The brain is damaged, to be sure, by the organic stress, be it poison, injury due to trauma, disease (as in encephalitis) or old age; but how the brain of the injured person reacts depends in a major way on the type of ego function which he had before the injury. Severe organic injury occurring in a person with previously effective ego functioning may cause great reduction of the ability of the brain to function without causing psychosis, whereas, in a person who previously had some type of defective ego, the injury may result in a severe organic psychosis. The hypothesis further implies that there is hope for psychological treatment of people with psychosis due to severe brain damage. If the ego which remains can be assisted toward more effective functioning, the person can be helped to recover from an organic psychosis. Although his function would not be perfect, he would be in markedly better condition. Thus in the treatment of organic psychosis more is needed than medical therapy. Good treatment always requires the concurrent application of psychological therapies.

Functional Psychoses—Schizophrenia

These are the psychoses which have no known origin and therefore may be postulated to be of psychological cause. These psychoses may occur in people of any age—from children below the age of three years to adults in their seventies who develop a functional psychosis for the first time. In this book the term *schizophrenia* will be used sparingly because I do not feel that it is a useful term. Almost all patients in a mental hospital are labeled one of several varieties of schizophrenic, as if this were a meaningful or helpful term.

Actually it groups together large numbers of extremely dissimilar patients, and further implies that a person so labeled will be hard to treat. If the patient is so unfortunate that he has this disease long enough for it to be labeled chronic schizophrenia, his chances for help are slim. He is often shuffled to a back ward where he is tolerated, not treated, his opportunity for help greatly diminished by the very label put on him.

Schizophrenic (*schizo* split; *phren* mind) may be meaningful in some cases in the sense that part of the patient's ego is in contact with reality and part or most is not, but it is not meaningful in the usual sense that the ego is split or shattered. The argument of what schizophrenia is has little merit because of the ambiguity of this widely used term. Nevertheless the very process of labeling is bad with psychotic people for when we label, we begin to think in stereotypes —to group them as if they were all alike. Because we do not understand them, we, with the use of labels, fall into the trap of thinking unrealistically even as they think. Although these terms will continue to be used, as will many psychiatric terms, they are poor because they may do harm to the patient.

We must think of psychotic people as human beings with the same needs as all others, living in the same world in which we live. Their difficulty is that they have a type of defective ego functioning which has caused them to shrink from the world into their own ego. They are still unique human beings whose only correct label is their own name. They must be given the respect of not being lumped into a group as a kind of "schiz," the slang term unfortunately often used among insensitive people who deal with these patients. This respect is vital, because these people are under the control of others: courts, psychiatrists, aides, etc. Having lost their freedom, they cannot defend themselves against an incorrect or potentially harmful label. If they get poor treatment because of a label, they suffer needlessly. In contrast, if a neurotic patient is labeled, he at least is still under his own initiative, and he may do something to escape the harm which might be caused by a label.

Before discussing specific types of psychosis, one point must be made clear. Psychoses are generally classified into two main groups, the acute psychoses and the chronic psychoses. In the usually accepted psychiatric sense, acute means that the psychotic behavior started within one year period prior to being severe enough to warrant psychiatric care. Chronic psychosis continues more or less unchanged from one year to a lifetime. Rather than use these arbitrary terms it is better to understand that the psychotic process is acute as long as the disease is going on actively.

To clarify in terms of ego function what is meant by active psychotic process: an active process is one in which the rigid or set, thickened pattern of the ego has not yet solidified completely. The ego, still in flux, has areas which are actively attempting to contact reality. Continuing to fight the rigidifying process which is changing his ego, the person fears the loss of contact with reality. This fear is, however, opposed by the fear of closeness which is driving him to break with the world. The battle is fought with the parts of the ego which are still intact. If he wins this battle he may have only a brief acute psychotic episode; if he loses, assuming no therapeutic intervention, he will gradually become a chronic, unchanging psychotic patient. Although the process may be short in time, as soon as the person loses complete contact he may be regarded as chronic.

Sometimes the fight between keeping in contact with reality and the withdrawal into the psychotic substitute within the ego ends in a draw. We may see this process going on for years unless something happens to turn the tide one way or another. As long as the process continues actively, the psychosis should be judged as acute. In psychosis, therefore, the person is caught between two opposing fears, one that he is going to lose contact with reality, the other that it seems so dangerous to remain in contact with the real world.

If he develops a psychosis, his needs suffer permanent loss of real satisfaction, but if he remains in the world he will have to continue close relationships with people whom he cannot tolerate because he is so frightened of his feelings in these relationships. Acute functional psychosis exists as long as the process is still evolving. Chronic psychosis occurs when we judge that the process has been resolved by a break with reality.

Functional Psychoses (Schizophrenia)

There are at least four main types of functional psychoses which are recognized. These include the paranoid psychosis (paranoid schizophrenia), catatonic psychosis (catatonic schizophrenia), hebephrenic psychosis (hebephrenic schizophrenia), and simple psychosis (simple schizophrenia). Another type is undifferentiated psychosis, in which no clear-cut differentiating symptoms exist. This is probably the most common diagnosis for people who have been psychotic for many years.

Types of Functional Psychoses

The type of functional psychosis is determined by how the psychotic person adjusts to his psychological environment. That is, when the thickened ego becomes a substitute for reality, the kind of reality it provides determines the type of psychotic reaction. There are many different ways in which the ego can do this job, some of which involve a seemingly incomplete break with reality.

In one large group of psychoses (paranoid) the break with reality may appear to be only partial, or in a certain area, whereas in other areas the ego may seem to be in good contact with reality. Probably, however, this seemingly good contact with reality is not true contact, but a type of psychotic contact which occurs only because the person feels safe now that he is psychotic. This apparent contact is the main source of difficulty in working with these patients because, although they may seem quite rational, they are still psychotic. If we are fooled into thinking them well we may discharge them, only to see a little later that they are far from cured. It is as if the psychosis is a safe den or lair into which they can always retreat, although, especially in the hospital, they may spend much of their time out in the world around the den. They are not cured of their psychosis, however, until they come to the conclusion that it is safe to stay out in the world without fleeing back into the den where their own ego becomes the substitute for reality.

Another part of the psychotic process which differentiates the psychotic types needs to be understood before describing the types in detail. This is the process of psychotic restitution, the actual way in which the psychotic person builds and develops the new world which exists in his own ego.

The process is the emergence of the psychotic character, the final solution to his problems, in his own ego. In this solution we observe the really crazy behavior, the hallucinations, the delusions, the catatonic postures, or the hebephrenic laughter. While this restitution continues, the person may relate to reality, but it is a restitutive relation to reality which masks the psychosis.

This restitutive contact with reality signifies a resolution of forces within the ego and must be differentiated from actual remission from the psychosis. *Restitution is a means of establishing equilibrium within the psychotic ego.* Because the ego is no longer torn by the fight between psychosis and reality, the restituted patient may seem to be more sane, though actually he is more psychotic. How he restitutes or how his psychotic character stabilizes determines the actual type of psychosis which we label. Again, however, this label is much less important than understanding the ego mechanism involved.

Paranoid Psychosis (Paranoid Schizophrenia)

In this psychosis the symptoms are primarily mental, with any psychotic physical activity secondary to psychotic thought and perception. The paranoid patient has retreated from the world to build himself a new and safer world, usually complete with hallucinations, delusions, and fixed ideas. He has masked his fear-produced hostile feelings against the world by a massive, psychotic use of projection. He says, "It is not I who am crazy, but rather the world. I'm okay and if you will only listen to my side you will see that the world is all wrong." He has solved his problems by stating that the one true world is the world of his ego, even though in a distorted way he recognizes his break with reality.

Rationalizing and projecting his belief that reality is wrong but he is right, he restitutes with hallucinations, delusions, fixed ideas, and psychotic obsessions and compulsions, all of which reinforce his position. He is not always comfortable, however, because his ego is not able to protect him completely. Thus even his own world, in which he may hear threatening voices, may be quite unsatisfactory. These voices are his own hostile feelings being reflected within his ego, which is unable to modify them.

With all his psychotic thought difficulties he is usually still able to carry on the routine of the hospital. He is the patient who, cooperative and giving little trouble, is able to do much work in the hospital. A paranoid patient is physically dangerous only if, in the process of fighting his psychotic process, he feels that someone wants to hurt him. Dangerous action may also occur if the restitution to his psychotic world is so unsatisfactory that out of desperation he strikes out hostilely. Although these cases are usually widely publicized, physically aggressive behavior is extremely rare. The paranoid patient is difficult to treat because in most cases he has restituted almost completely; thus he is set in his psychosis.

Catatonic

The catatonic patient has restituted also, but his restitution includes not only mental symptoms but also physical symptoms. His whole body is involved in his psychosis. Often mute and inactive, he may assume bizarre postures or attitudes for years during which time he is almost totally psychotic. His ego has taken over his body as well as his mind so that he is almost physically bound into his catatonic psychosis. These patients are extremely resistant to treatment because the exceedingly thick-walled, closely bound ego has produced a nearly completely psychotic character.

Hebephrenic

The hebephrenic, seen less frequently than the paranoid or catatonic, still exists in substantial numbers in most hospitals. In his psychotic restitution he has been able to make his psychosis gay and happy, so that he is characterized as a mental clown. Laughing inappropriately at everything, he seems to enjoy his psychosis. For unknown reasons, perhaps because he does not have sufficient ego strength to be paranoid or catatonic, he takes the course that psychosis is a wonderful place for him. He again is very difficult to treat, for he is not unhappy as he is.

Simple Psychosis

The patient designated as a simple schizophrenic or a simple psychotic, does not have the thick ego requisite for psychosis as that term is used herein. Rather, he is a person with an ego weakness so extreme that often he has no ego at all. Having long since given up any emotions or ego reactions, he attempts little in the way of ego functioning, existing with no particular drives and no particular attempts to relate to the world. Without enough ego to be crazy or neurotic, he might be classified under the generalized ego weakness discussed in Chapter 12.

He is not detached from reality, nor has he created a new reality within his ego. He is the bum, wino, or skid row character who drifts along, barely existing. Although some of these people are placed in mental hospitals because they cannot take care of themselves, most live a skid row existence supported by missions. The term simple psychosis or simple schizophrenia is a misnomer and should be dropped. This diagnosis is retained only by those who think it necessary to diagnose these socially dependent patients as some type of schizophrenic.

Undifferentiated Psychosis

Patients classified as undifferentiated psychotics make up the largest single group in any hospital. Although they do not fit into any of the three main categories, they obviously are living within the world of their own ego. These patients often exhibit symptoms or behavior typical of one of the three classes, but as time goes on they seem to fit less into any particular category. This lack of specific symptoms again underscores the importance of recognizing the type of ego defect involved rather than its particular manifestations. Patients who have rigid, fixed, thickened egos are psychotic; the problem is to help them toward a more effective ego, not to concern ourselves with their symptoms or behavior.

Childhood Psychosis

Psychosis is not unknown in childhood although the majority of psychotic people develop the characteristic thickened ego between adolescence and the age of forty-five. In early childhood it is difficult to tell whether a psychosis is present or not because the child lives normally in a world partly of his own choosing. Whereas we do not think it is unusual for a child of two to five to have an imaginary companion some of the time, if the child prefers his companion to reality at all times, he is bordering on psychosis.

Such a child may indulge in bizarre and peculiar behavior, exhibit odd body movements, twirl or continually walk on his toes, and make only a feeble effort to contact reality. The psychotic child seems content with isolation from reality, talks his own often unintelligible language, has peculiar eating habits, and may refuse to become bowel-trained. None of these symptoms, if isolated, indicates psychosis, but when a child has many of them and, in addition, is only in limited contact with reality, the diagnosis may well be childhood psychosis. These severe problems require early special treatment. In many cases it seems as if the child's ego were unable to begin to make the relationship to his mother and others which are the necessary beginnings of contact with reality. Often he has healthy siblings and parents who are, for the most part, quite adequate.

What causes children to take this course? Much research is being done to find out. Childhood psychosis, starting sometimes in infancy, seems in many cases to be a congenital ego defect. Although there is some evidence for this thesis at the present time, it certainly should not be used to explain why the majority of psychotic patients develop their psychosis.

17

Depression and Psychosomatic Disease

THIS CHAPTER COMPLETES THE PART OF THE BOOK DEVOTED to abnormal or defective ego functioning. Although depression and psychosomatic disease are dissimilar in appearance, they involve essentially the same ego mechanism. This is the mechanism of depression, which was described briefly under the ego reactions in Chapter 4 of Part I.

In depression the principal difficulty lies in the inability of the ego to handle angry feelings satisfactorily. Normally, anger is discharged harmlessly into the world in a myriad of different ways, each of which helps the ego to unburden itself of the anger. In depression and psychosomatic illness, because of fear of loss of love, fear of retaliation, or the removal of the object of the anger, the ego is unable to discharge angry emotions. The result is that the anger remains within the ego where it exerts a harmful influence in either of two ways.

1. The anger can stay in the ego, enveloping and immobilizing it so that it becomes nonfunctional, producing a depression.
2. The anger can be rejected by the ego pathologically and discharged inwardly to the body where it attaches itself to some vulnerable organ or organ system, producing a psychosomatic disease.

In each case it is the inability of the ego to handle angry emotion effectively which precipitates the illness. In some cases people alternate between depression and psychosomatic disease. This condition, which will be described later, is important because it demonstrates that if anger builds up to a point where it cannot be expressed to the outside world, it either envelops and immobilizes the ego or is discharged through an organ or organ system with resultant psychosomatic disease.

Depression

Depression may exist in all degrees of severity, from a simple, week-long mild depressed state which only moderately hampers the individual's functioning to a severe, psychotic depression requiring hospitalization. The severity of the depression is determined by two factors:

1. The amount of the anger which cannot be discharged into the world.
2. The strength of the ego of the depressed person.

Thus a person with a weak ego may become greatly depressed with only a moderate amount of ego-contained anger, whereas a person with a strong ego might be able to hold much more anger and yet be less depressed.

It is fundamental in the history of depressed people that they encounter a specific situation in which they lose something or someone representing a strong psychological attachment. It is also characteristic that the situation in which they suffer this loss is one which they can do little or nothing about. An example is the commonly occurring depression or grief which usually follows the death of a loved person.

Although many people find it difficult to believe that a depressed, grief-stricken person is angry, this is actually the case. He is angry at being separated from his loved one, as a child might be angry when Mother leaves him with a baby sitter. The adult, however, cannot effectively express this anger because the person at whom it is directed is dead. Along with the anger within the ego of the depressed person which arises when he is "deserted" by the death of his loved one there is the inability to cope with this strong emotion. Because a person is expected to show any emotion except anger after the death of a loved one, the anger is difficult to express. Normally, it is discharged during the period of mourning, a socially and psychologically acceptable method of sublimating anger. Thus, as the process of mourning comes to an end, the depression usually lifts.

In those cases where depression continues, however, the relationship between the depressed person and the deceased loved one was too close. The depressed person was so dependent on the deceased that he may have resented his dependence. An example of this one-way relationship is that which exists between an overprotective mother and her child. The anger may never leave the depressed person because death has now destroyed any possibility for him to resolve the one-way relationship. Long term, sometimes permanent, depression results.

Depression may also occur when a person loses something or someone symbolically, as in the case of a parent whose child grows up and no longer needs the parental ministrations. Thus, in a symbolic sense, his child is lost. Among orthodox Jews when a member of the family marries outside the faith, the miscreant is considered dead. The family goes through a symbolic funeral and mourning period which serves to express the anger caused by this religious desertion.

Often the depressed person talks of suicide because he feels empty and worthless due to the anger which has immobilized his ego. When the ego is restricted in carrying out its necessary functions, the ego reaction—depression—is accompanied by feelings of worthlessness and self-deprecation. During these periods of self-deprecation, the depressed person may attempt to destroy himself, thus emphasizing in a dramatic way his sense of worthlessness. He is often made more depressed by the sympathy his state arouses in others. The more compassion he receives, the worse he feels because it is not easy to express the trapped anger in the face of well-meaning friends.

An extremely depressed person, therefore, may commit suicide because his ego is so burdened with hostile, self-attacking anger that he concludes death is preferable to the misery of his depressed state. Thus, it is not unusual for a depressed person to commit suicide in order to completely remove the anger from his ego—a final irrational solution to his problem. Suicide usually occurs before or after the *depth* of the depression because during the period of greatest intensity he is too immobilized to do anything. He may kill himself either before the most severe depression in anticipation of the misery to come, or afterwards to avoid repeating the suffering experienced previously during the intense period of depression. Therefore, suicide comes not, as might be anticipated, while the depressed person is "sick," but often unexpectedly, when everyone feels that he is well on the way to recovery.

The ego, however, has an alternative to suicide: psychosis. When the feeling of depression becomes so strong that the ego is overwhelmingly immobilized by the entrapped anger, it reacts by forming a wall within itself against the anger. The ego wall, however, separates the person not only from the anger, but also from reality, so that he becomes psychotic. In this state he may or may not be successful in venting the anger. If he is successful he may become manic, with the extreme flexibility of ego so characteristic of mania. Reaching the pinnacle of psychological omnipotence, in this psychosis, he has no bounds, no restrictions on his ego at all. Mania or manic psychosis was much more common fifty years ago than it is today, though the reasons for its decline are not clear.

If the depressed psychotic is unsuccessful in venting his anger, he will suffer the horrible alternative of being extremely depressed as well as psychotic. Withdrawn and often bizarre, he still suffers severe depression. At this time he may commit suicide with the psychotic logic that he is revenging himself against the lost object or person. Which course he takes depends upon his ego organization and his prior ego strength. What the lost person or object meant to him and other factors are not usually known, although they may be understood in some cases after study by a psychiatrist.

Finally, it must be noted that not all the causes of deep depression are unrealistic as they appear in the examples given above. It is quite possible to be dependent upon another person economically, socially, or for status, and to be realistically rejected by that person. The boss who snubs a faithful long-term subordinate by appointing his own son to the coveted vice-presidency often precipitates depression in the subordinate. This is an example of a situation which few people can handle successfully. In this case, for the subordinate to vent his anger at his boss is an economic impossibility so he may become depressed until he can extricate himself from his predicament. Unfortunately, being depressed, he is in poor condition to help himself. In fact, a feature of our "organization society" is never to hope for anything too much so that you never have to get depressed. The price paid by the organization man for this type of existence (sans hope) is obvious.

The treatment of depression, one of the few psychiatric conditions for which there is a definite therapy, is in many cases specific. It is discussed in some detail in Part III.

Psychosomatic Disease

More and more medical conditions are being diagnosed as psychosomatic, that is, an organic disease caused by psychological factors. It must be clearly differentiated from two separate conditions in which there is *no* organic disease or tissue damage: hysteria or conversion reactions where there is loss of function, and hypochondriasis, where there is no loss of function although the person is neurotically convinced that organic disease is present.

There is nothing imaginary about psychosomatic diseases, however; they are serious and can be fatal. Although the cause may be psychological, the result is organic. Duodenal ulcer, a psychosomatic disease, is a sore, raw, ulcerated area in the bowel just below the stomach which can be complicated by bleeding or perforation. If the disease is not speedily and properly treated when these serious complications occur, the result can be fatal. It should also be understood immediately that the treatment of psychosomatic disease is both psychiatric and medical. Although the word psychosomatic is not the most descriptive term that could be applied to this disease—it does not emphasize sufficiently the real tissue damage involved—it is so widely used and accepted that it is continued here.

The cause of psychosomatic disease has already been briefly mentioned in the beginning of this section. To elaborate further, however, the ego of the person involved has found a way to channel anger from his ego into his body. At the price of severe disease, even in the face of death, his ego continues to channel the anger in this direction. These people develop an ego which usually functions rather well, and to all appearances anger is one of the emotions they are best able to handle. Even when they are extremely ill they are often capable of taking almost anything with a smile. In periods when they are uncomfortable but not seriously ill, however, they are often quite opposite: irascible and angry. In trying to dissipate the anger, they are not usually successful.

When well, this type of person is smiling, willing, and hard-working, but he is always vulnerable to psychosomatic illness even while smiling. He is efficient, prompt, orderly, and gets along well with others. Although all the angry emotions which arise from the realities of life seem to be taken in stride, actually they are channeled into the person's particular psychosomatic pathway instead of being expressed. Eventually the organ involved breaks down and disease occurs.

This leads to another feature of psychosomatic disease, its waxing and waning characteristic. Severe attacks are followed by a period of healing. When intense anger is channeled inward the severe attacks occur; when anger is dissipated in the attack or in some other better way, the disease lessens. There are cases when the person receives psychiatric help which ordinarily would alleviate the disease but the illness continues, perhaps fatally. This occurs when tissue damage is so severe that the normal recuperative powers of the body are unable to stop the decline. Ulcerative colitis, for example, sometimes takes this course.

Persons with psychosomatic disease are usually resistant to psychiatric treatment because they do not accept the psychiatric implications of their illness, and "to prove it" they point out their diseased organ or organs. Unfortunately, many patients are reinforced in their beliefs by attending physicians or surgeons who also do not understand or accept the psychological causes of these conditions, and who therefore treat only the medical aspect. This problem is discussed in Part III.

When patients with psychosomatic disease are treated medically or surgically by powerful drugs and/or radical operations, the organic but not the psychological part of the disease is often greatly helped. Unfortunately, in many cases this type of treatment acts as a barrier against the old way of channeling anger. The organ where the anger previously was discharged is either strengthened by the anti-stress drugs, such as cortisone, or it is absent, having been removed surgically. Now the anger must stay within the ego, at least until it can find another outlet, so that, to the dismay and concern of everyone, the patient becomes extremely depressed. He may even be suicidal. It is always dangerous, therefore, to treat these diseases radically without an understanding of their psychiatric implications.

There is a psychiatric theory as to why people develop a particular psychosomatic disease. The theory postulates that these people have a certain character type combined with an organ predisposed to breakdown under psychological stress. For example: According to the theory a person with a stomach weakness, who develops excess acid in his stomach, is prone to stomach ulcer; and also, the ulcer patient has a basically dependent, though outwardly driving personality —he is angry because he must submerge his dependent needs. This same character and conflict, however, seem to exist in all psychosomatic conditions and many others. There is at present no good theoretical explanation for the occurrence of psychosomatic disease in one site vs. another.

Specific Psychosomatic Conditions

A note of caution must precede the discussion of specific psychosomatic diseases. It is necessary that care be used in interpreting what is psychosomatic and what is not. All diseases, from the common cold to cancer, are influenced by psychological factors. In most diseases, however, there are definite and known factors which are not psychological in origin; for example, an infecting virus in polio. It is not the purpose of this book to discuss how all diseases are affected or possibly affected by psychological factors. Nevertheless, it should be understood that anything which tends to weaken ego functioning will in turn be detrimental to any medical condition, be it a broken leg or chicken pox.

Conversely, anything which tends to strengthen ego functioning has a beneficial affect on any disease. Medical care rendered by a competent physician is always ego strengthening. While it is true that the psychological factors arising in any disease must be recognized and dealt with, beyond the general conditions are the very important but more limited major psychosomatic diseases. These diseases are discussed individually in the following pages.

Peptic Ulcer—Stomach Ulcer—Duodenal Ulcer

This is a disease of the upper part of the gastrointestinal tract. Much evidence has accumulated which indicates that people with peptic ulcer are constantly digesting, continually secreting excessive acid in the stomach. Under the stress of the anger turned inward this excess acid breaks through the normal protective mucous barrier of the bowel and forms a peptic ulcer, usually in the duodenum, occasionally in the stomach. Over the years the process of an ulcer developing and healing may repeat itself many times within the susceptible patient. All the complications of stomach ulcer may occur in such cases, making this disease difficult and protracted in treatment.

Because there is no known organic cause of this disease, the treatment of choice in severe cases should be psychiatric as well as medical. In mild cases, where an ulcer occurs and then quickly heals, consultation with a competent, understanding medical doctor may be sufficient. In these cases there is no need for immediate psychiatric treatment unless other psychiatric conditions are present, such as the healing ulcer leaving the patient severely depressed. Psychiatric referral should be made when the condition is severe and persistent, or when a referring physician, perceiving emotional difficulties in the patient, can use the ulcer as a wedge to encourage the patient to get help.

Ileitis, Colitis (Ulcerative or Mucous or Spastic)

There are many pathological conditions of the middle and lower bowel which result in serious medical complications. Unlike upper bowel disease, such as peptic ulcer, these conditions rarely heal quickly or easily and often develop complications severe enough to necessitate surgery. Probably no case of ileitis in the history of medicine received more publicity than President Eisenhower's, which was so serious that surgery was required. As in ulcer, there is no organic cause for the disease. If it recurs after surgery or steadily becomes worse, psychiatric help is necessary, for this illness can be fatal if not checked. Although the psychotherapeutic treatment again is difficult and may fail to halt the course of the disease, it is, together with good medical care, the best course.

Asthma

Although some types of asthma in children are allergic or partially allergic in origin, adult asthma is often a psychosomatic disease because emotional stress precipitates attacks and no allergic or other organic cause can be found. Patients almost never die during asthma attacks or directly from asthma, but the patients' lungs are so stretched that death may result from chronic lung disease which originated from severe asthma.

Asthma is a particularly frightening disease because the most important physiologic need—the need for air—is directly blocked. Whereas there are literally scores of different ways of treating asthma, psychiatric treatment ranks far down the list in frequency of use. Rarely is a psychiatrist consulted until severe secondary lung damage occurs. Even if the psychiatrist can help at this point, the permanent lung damage remains. In asthma which does not quickly respond to medical treatment a psychiatrist should be consulted. Often early psychiatric treatment coupled with good medical management is the only satisfactory course of treatment.

Urticaria or Giant Hives

This condition which usually occurs as brief, severe attacks, can be a chronic condition in which the patient suffers almost continually from hives. Although this extremely baffling condition rarely endangers life or causes permanent tissue damage, it can be seriously incapacitating. If the allergic swelling attacks the larynx, the air passage can be abruptly closed, necessitating quick treatment to prevent suffocation. Extremely resistant to medical care, urticaria rarely receives psychiatric care because the usually acute and brief process is over before either patient or physician feels impelled to call a psychiatrist. Probably in the chronic cases, or even where severe attacks are frequent, psychiatric intervention is indicated.

Eczema

This chronic skin condition is not only closely related to hives but also intimately related to depression. In periods where their skin is cleared by the use of drugs, eczema patients are often depressed. They derive immense satisfaction in scratching, almost angrily attacking their bodies, during which time depression is absent. They are preoccupied with skin and skin satisfactions. Because they respond poorly to dermatologic treatment, they are often referred to psychiatrists for help. Although psychiatric treatment is sometimes quite beneficial, the psychiatrist must be prepared for a long, difficult therapy.

Migraine Headache

Migraine is a severe headache always limited to one side of the head at one time, though the affected side may shift. In severe cases nausea, vomiting, and visual disturbances occur. The blood vessels on the affected side of the skull, scalp, and probably the brain, are constricted. Often in this process some permanent changes are wrought in the blood vessels of the affected side, but except for this there are none of the major tissue changes seen in the other psychosomatic conditions. Nevertheless, because this disease is neither hysterical nor hypochondriacal, it should be classed as psychosomatic.

Although there is no known cause for this disease, there are some excellent medical therapies which will relieve individual attacks. Patients rarely seek psychiatric help because the headaches are usually over quickly and because while they are well they do not have the motivation to see a psychiatrist. In many cases the headaches are severe enough to be crippling, and medical therapies fail. In these cases a psychiatrist should be consulted, for psychiatric treatment is often effective.

Other Diseases

There are many diseases about which there is debate at the present time concerning whether or not they are psychosomatic. An example is high blood pressure, or essential hypertension. It is my opinion that the six diseases discussed above constitute the major psychosomatic illnesses, with others still subject to speculation and requiring better proof. Actually, even for the six diseases mentioned, there are many who say that even these are not really psychosomatic. They point both to the lack of proof and to the difficulty that psychiatrists, "for all their talk," have in treating these illnesses. In this field of medicine, in which opinions are much more widespread than facts, it is imperative that everyone keep his mind receptive to new information whether or not it is compatible with a preconceived opinion.

III

PSYCHIATRIC TREATMENT

Introduction

PART III OF THIS BOOK ENCOMPASSES THE SUBJECT OF PSYchiatric treatment. To cover this subject fully all of its components are discussed, including the people who treat, the problems of treatment, and the various treatments available. In order to avoid certain misunderstandings about treatment, especially about its *effectiveness and reliability,* it is necessary to introduce the subject with a brief discussion of these aspects of the process.

Psychiatric treatment means the active participation by a psychiatrist in some type of therapeutic program which results in more effective ego functioning in the patient. In psychiatry, as in the rest of medicine, the effectiveness of this participation is difficult to assess. For example, two patients apply to a psychiatric clinic with similar problems. One is accepted for treatment, one is placed on the clinic waiting list. When, after six months, the person on the waiting list is contacted, he says that he is much better and that he no longer desires help. The person in treatment continues for another six months before being discharged as improved. It is evident that ego strengthening took place in both cases, though by any acceptable definition only one received psychiatric treatment.

In another case a patient is committed to a large state mental hospital where he receives minimal care for two years until he is discharged as improved. Certainly by definition this, too, is psychiatric treatment, but actually there was only proximity to a psychiatric situation. In another case a psychiatrist reports a patient in treatment who never spoke during the therapy hour. Relatives, however, reported great improvement.

There is also the great puzzle of what happens to the large numbers who call clinics, apply for hospital care, or have one brief interview with a psychiatric worker and then are never heard from again. What happens to these people? Do they languish with permanently defective egos or do they eventually achieve better functioning? That they do not continue to ask for help indicates that many improve without any definite psychiatric care. Finally, much of what at present passes for psychiatric treatment tends to increase the ego defects of the patient. Often subtle in individual therapy, in hospital care poor treatment is at times blatant. In many of our huge, crowded mental hospitals those who receive benefit often do so in spite of the treatment; there are many, however, who become more ego defective, more severely psychotic as their nontherapeutic incarceration is prolonged over the years. Therefore, in psychiatry as in the rest of medicine two facts must be recognized:

1. Much healing takes place without benefit of therapist or therapy.
2. Treatment does not necessarily lead to improvement; in fact, in some situations, just the opposite occurs.

This part of the book details what are believed to be the important elements of good psychiatric treatment, treatment which should lead to improvement in the patients' ego functioning. This does not imply that all of the problems of defective ego functioning can be solved by even the best treatment programs. Indeed, there is some question whether or not it is desirable to increase therapy facilities drastically even though there seems to be such great need. This question arises because the number of people who need help will always exceed any treatment capacity unless some effective program of mental hygiene can be instituted.

Perhaps it would be more expedient to spend greater effort toward making it easier for more people to develop effective egos rather than to increase facilities for help. At present such a program is difficult to initiate because of fear and ignorance of psychiatry and its connection with mental illness, a situation similar to that which once existed among those who fought sanitation when cholera and dysentery were rife. The dissemination of knowledge has solved many "insoluble" problems, so that it seems certain that increased understanding will lead to many more effective egos than will any program of psychiatric treatment, although this phase of medicine will continue to grow in scope and importance.

18

❖

The People Who Treat

PSYCHIATRISTS

PSYCHIATRISTS ARE MEDICAL DOCTORS WHO HAVE RECEIVED specific training in psychiatry after they have completed a four-year course in medicine and one year of internship. Working with patients having all types of defective egos, they train for three years in hospitals and clinics under the supervision of more experienced psychiatrists who also instruct them in psychiatric theory. In addition, psychiatrists have at least several months of training in neurology, a branch of medicine which deals with organic diseases of the nervous system. There is no prerequisite that psychiatrists be trained in the humanities, in psychology, or in sociology, although their work is directly related to these fields. In the practice of psychotherapy very little detailed medical knowledge is used, though in the treatment of some patients, such as those suffering from hysteria, hypochondriasis or psychosomatic disease, medical knowledge is valuable. Medical knowledge is vital in administering electric shock treatments, a speciality of psychiatrists in urban centers.

Psychiatrists may elect to train further and become psychoanalysts, a group who practice a certain very rigidly defined, specific form of psychotherapy started by Sigmund Freud. This additional training takes from three to ten years beyond the regular three-year psychiatric training. Much popular confusion exists concerning the difference between a psychiatrist and a psychoanalyst. Briefly, a psychoanalyst is almost always a psychiatrist, but a psychiatrist need not become a psychoanalyst unless he has a bent toward practicing the specific type of therapy called psychoanalysis.

Psychiatric Social Workers

These people, who have had extensive undergraduate training in psychology and sociology, train in graduate status and obtain a Master's Degree from an approved professional school of social science. They may even go further and earn a Doctor of Philosophy degree in their field. Social workers are trained to treat people with all types of ego defects. Although usually employed in public agencies, it is not unusual for them to be in private practice, working either with a psychiatrist or by themselves. Their training, though somewhat different from that of the psychiatrist, is likewise directed toward treating persons with defective egos. They have extensive theoretical knowledge in dealing with human problems because of their study of sociology and psychology, and are often better grounded in these subjects than psychiatrists. Usually they lack the intensive training in psychotherapy that psychiatrists receive, but they have much more training and experience in working with the family and environment of the patient. Thus, by trying to alleviate bad social environments they treat both the person and the world in which he lives.

Although social workers have less status than psychiatrists, they are still well qualified to help in the treatment of the mentally ill. They lack status, not because they have an inferior education but because they do not have medical training, an extremely high status symbol in our society. Social workers function in all social agencies, in institutions of all types, in general hospitals, and as parole and probation officers.

Clinical Psychologists

Rising into prominence after World War II, this relatively new profession suffers because at present it has neither the status of psychiatry nor the tradition of social work. Nevertheless, it is making rapid progress and some of the most skilled workers in the field of mental illness are to be found among the clinical psychologists. Their training begins with four years of undergraduate work emphasizing psychology, math, and science. In graduate school, where the Doctor of Philosophy degree is earned, emphasis is placed on research in the motivating factors behind normal and abnormal human behavior, and on the construction and administration of tests to assess ego functioning. Until recently clinical psychologists were less intensively trained than psychiatrists in the actual treatment of people with defective egos because only limited facilities were open to them. Now, however, more opportunities for training in treatment are available.

Because of the pressing load of patients who need treatment, the Veterans' Administration and state hospitals are using this newer group and providing additional training and job facilities for psychologists to work with the mentally ill. Though more hospitals and clinics now accept them, many people still think that clinical psychologists, no matter how well trained, are not able to treat patients with defective egos except under direct psychiatric supervision. Many psychologists, however, can and do treat patients without psychiatric supervision, often maintaining private offices for this purpose. There is danger because laws against people setting up practice with little or no training are still weak, and in fact, in few states is the public properly protected against charlatans who may call themselves clinical psychologists.

There are many problems to be solved before clinical psychologists gain a secure niche in the field of treating mental illness; nevertheless many of the best clinicians in the country are clinical psychologists whose help in treating patients is needed and welcome.

Psychiatric Nurses

In mental hospitals the psychiatric nurse has the brunt of the responsibility for the everyday welfare and progress of the patient. She is a graduate nurse who has received from one to three years of special training. Much of the good treatment in institutions for the mentally ill is due to the nurses. They supervise the psychiatric technicians and their cooperation is important in creating and maintaining the therapeutic atmosphere so vital to good hospital treatment.

Psychiatric Technicians

Psychiatric technicians work directly with the patients in a mental hospital. Over ninety per cent of the contact that patients have with personnel is with the psychiatric technician. Usually with high school but not college training, their pay is low and the work, if they are conscientious, is hard. Most of their training comes from the professional staff of the hospital, so that the quality of treatment they give the patients depends upon the type of training and cooperation they receive from the professional staff. Although they have little job status, they can and should be given personal status through praise and cooperation from the psychiatrists in charge of the hospital. If they do not receive this attention, the patients under their care will receive only custody, or even, in unfortunate instances, maltreatment.

Supervisors, Counselors, Guards, Etc.

These custody people make up the staff of institutions for adult and juvenile delinquents. Often with some college training or a college degree, they have much more status than psychiatric technicians, and in many cases receive good pay. The essential functions of this staff, the key part of any custodial institution, is discussed in detail later. In addition to some college courses in psychology and sociology that they usually have taken, they should also receive active training within both the institution and its parent organization. For example, the California Youth Authority, which cares for institutionalized delinquents, has an active in-service training program for all employees. This institutional training is vital because universities do not provide the specialized training needed. People who stay at college long enough to receive extensive training usually go into administration rather than into direct work with institution inmates.

This, then, comprises the main list of those who treat. The field is still rife with petty professional jealousies and status problems which do not augur well for utilizing each person in his most needed position. Duplication of work between professional groups results in less treatment than could be available in already overcrowded facilities. There is bickering about who should do what and who is qualified to do what. In the highly organized psychiatric clinic a psychiatrist interviews the patient, a social worker interviews his family, and a psychologist tests and diagnoses the patient. The information is then presented to the chief psychiatrist who decides, usually without ever seeing the patient, whether or not the applicant will be accepted for treatment. This is a cumbersome and time-wasting procedure. Much better is the procedure in smaller, less organized clinics where everyone treats, where discussions are held to solve problems, not to rehash old issues, and where status is subordinate to the welfare of the patient.

19
❖
The Types of Psychiatric Treatment

THERE ARE TWO MAIN SUBDIVISIONS OF PSYCHIATRIC TREATment: psychological treatments, which include psychotherapy, and the physical–chemical treatments, which include drug, shock, and the surgical treatments. In this book, which deals primarily with the ego, psychological treatment is stressed,

Psychological Treatments

Individual Psychotherapy

This is the best known of all psychological treatments. As popularly conceived, the patient and the therapist discuss the patient's problems privately. Treatment is done in clinics, offices, and, to some extent, in institutions. Individual psychotherapy usually takes place on a regular basis, one to six times a week, the usual session lasting approximately fifty minutes. In practice, good therapy usually is done on a one, two, or three-times-a-week schedule.

Some psychiatrists, usually psychoanalysts, see selected patients four to six times a week. Contrary to popular opinion, the additional sessions do not necessarily mean better therapy or "deeper" therapy. How helpful therapy is to the patient depends on his ego strength and the capability of the psychiatrist far more than on the type or the frequency of treatment. Therefore, a patient with only a moderately defective ego is able to benefit from the relationship with the psychiatrist far more than the patient who has an extremely defective ego. The question of the "depth" of the therapy is meaningless. It is interesting to hear both lay and trained people discuss therapy, saying that a certain psychiatrist does "deep" therapy or that another one doesn't. As will be explained later, psychotherapy is only one thing. If it works at all to help the patient develop a more effective ego, it is "deep" therapy. If it doesn't work, it can be as "deep as the ocean" with no benefit to the patient. "Superficial" or "surface therapy" doesn't describe anything unless perhaps it conveys the meaning that the therapy is not effective.

The length of time a person sees a psychiatrist is variable. Usually, however, in one to two years the patient can make considerable progress toward a more effective ego. This time may seem excessive, but if the situation is considered realistically, it is not very long. It is possible for a thirty-five year old man with a defective ego to receive help from a psychiatrist seeing him only twice a week over a two-year period. This is two hundred hours to help an ego which after thirty-five years is still in the condition where psychiatric help is needed. The objective observer should reach the conclusion that the time required for help has been not excessive, but very short indeed.

Group Psychotherapy

Group psychotherapy has become widely used since World War II. Largely started in the armed services, it has now spread to include every place where psychotherapy is done. Office, clinic, and institution are all suitable sites for group therapy. Psychiatrists unfamiliar with this technique have in some cases tended to oppose this form of therapy, thus making it generally less accepted than individual treatment. Even where it is accepted it is usually with the reservation that it is only for people with mild ego defects. No reliable evidence supports these general statements about group therapy. It is a question of clinical judgment on the part of an unbiased therapist. Patients with all types of ego defects have been found to benefit from group as well as from individual therapy. In some cases they may be combined as, for example, in a schedule of one individual session and one group session each week.

There are a great many patients who seek care in clinics or private offices who would do as well in group therapy as in individual therapy. Although some cannot tolerate the group and need individual therapy, many others do better in group treatment. Group therapy is extremely valuable in institutions with a staff too small to give everyone individual therapy. The great advantage of group therapy is that one therapist can help at least five times as many patients as he could by devoting the same time and effort to individual therapy. Groups are usually made up of from five to eight patients.

In private practice group therapy is difficult to implement because patients do not come in large numbers at one time and because many of them are prejudiced against this treatment. The patient usually does not want to wait for four or five others so that a group can be formed, nor do new patients want to join a group in progress. In clinics and institutions this should be the therapy of choice for many patients because of the obvious saving of therapist time. If there is one immediate way to increase the time available to help people with no increase in cost, it is to increase the amount of group therapy being done. At present, I would estimate that, at most, ten per cent of all psychotherapy time is devoted to group therapy. If this figure were increased to only forty per cent (thinking in terms of six-person groups), the number of people presently being seen would double without the addition of one more therapist or facility. Even without definite proof of the effectiveness of group therapy, these figures should indicate the need to explore further this additional source of help. Certainly of the thousands of people who are denied clinic treatment, many would be willing to try group therapy rather than nothing. Still there is professional prejudice and public apathy, both based on unfamiliarity with the method. It is hoped that people who cannot afford the fee for private therapy, or who are denied individual therapy in clinics due to lack of time, will ask for group therapy.

Therapeutic Atmosphere—Institutional Therapy

In all psychotherapy, individual or group, there must exist a therapeutic atmosphere. In institutions the whole staff must work to create this atmosphere in order to increase the patient's ego strength. The principles of good psychotherapy are applied to a community of people to help the institutionalized group toward developing more effective egos. Without this atmosphere, institutions can only perform the service of removing the patient from the community. Under these conditions only a little haphazard therapy is possible in contrast to the large amount accomplished where a concerted planned, staff effort produces a therapeutic atmosphere.

Physical—Chemical—Therapies

Shock Treatments

In this treatment the patient is rendered unconscious, either by insulin or electricity and, while unconscious, he may have one or more severe convulsions. These convulsions are similar to those produced by an epileptic seizure. At the present time electricity is usually used, although a few places still use the older and much more dangerous insulin shock. There is no proved difference between the effect of insulin and electric shock; however, electric rather than insulin shock treatments are preferred because they are almost completely safe and only rarely cause complications. These treatments, used for a variety of conditions, at present appear to be most successful in the treatment of depression. Shock also helps some forms of psychosis, but in these cases it is far less predictable than in the treatment of depression. Many psychiatrists think that in institutions where a good therapeutic atmosphere exists shock should be reserved for either depressed people or people who have depression as a major feature of their psychosis.

Drugs—Chemicals

There is a whole armamentarium of psychiatric tranquilizing or energizing drugs and more are being produced daily. Huge sums of money are being spent to promote these drugs to physicians with claims that are extravagant, to say the least; hysterical, to say the most. Although these drugs do have a place, many reliable studies have shown that other factors besides the drugs have been responsible for progress which at first was attributed to them. These drugs can render people more comfortable, they can make a bad reality more tolerable, and they can often quiet an agitated or violent patient so that he can better utilize psychotherapy. Not miraculous in the sense penicillin was and is, nevertheless if used with good judgment they can help certain patients.

Tranquilizing drugs are used far more by non-psychiatric physicians than by psychiatrists in an attempt to help the very large numbers of medical patients who come to their offices with emotional problems. If they are either used indiscriminately or substituted for needed psychotherapy, as they often are now, the patient will suffer. Unfortunately, the reason behind the huge push by the drug companies toward marketing these drugs is far from altruistic; as a result both the conscientious non-psychiatric physician and the psychiatrist have become dismayed in their efforts to evaluate properly the therapeutic effects of the various drugs.

Surgery

A chapter on psychiatric treatment would not be complete without a short discussion of psycho-surgery or lobotomy. This procedure has now fallen into general disfavor and is relatively unused. Better hospital facilities, together with the increased acceptance of the therapeutic atmosphere, has generally reduced the need to employ this drastic procedure. Lobotomy was usually performed on psychiatric patients who were generally uncontrollable because of wild and aggressive behavior. It was found that severing the frontal lobe from the rest of the brain reduced or eliminated the wild emotions. The patient became tractable, but unfortunately his brain was so damaged that his recovery could proceed only so far, being limited by this severe surgical brain lesion. Now this form of control is available by the use of some of the powerful tranquilizing drugs in large doses and by better treatment of the psychotic patient. These alternate, and almost always preferable, methods of control have eliminated all but a very few lobotomies.

20

Problems Inherent in Psychiatric Treatment

Specific and General Aspects of Psychiatric Treatment

IN MOST FIELDS OF MEDICINE IT IS EASIER TO PRESCRIBE correct treatment than it is to make the correct diagnosis. If one can arrive at an accurate diagnosis, there are then certain treatments which are known to be best. This is not to imply that medical treatment is simple, but in medicine it is usually the diagnosis which presents the difficulties. For example, a man with a severe sore throat would receive penicillin if the diagnosis was a streptococcus infection localized in the throat. He would not be given penicillin by a competent physician if there was no indication to prove a bacteriological infection or if the physician diagnosed a virus-infected throat.

Also, in medicine there are diseases which defy diagnosis, such as a child with a high fever at night who is well and without fever in the morning. Speculation could proceed, but no diagnosis would be possible; furthermore, whether treatment was instituted or not, few doctors would lay the cure to the treatment. There are also diagnosed diseases for which there is no specific curative treatment. Examples are some of the leukemias in which treatment is at present palliative; we hope, however, that current research may soon lead to a definite treatment which either cures the disease or greatly prolongs life. Thus medicine is concerned primarily with diagnosis followed by the application of a specific treatment for specific disease.

In psychiatry the situation is entirely different. It would be excellent if, for a given type of defective ego, there was a given psychiatric treatment, but unfortunately this is not the case. Although there are several different types of psychiatric treatments, there is probably only one specific treatment which is applied to a specific condition. This is electric shock treatment for certain types of depression. The remaining bulk of psychiatric treatment, classified under psychotherapy, is nonspecific.

Psychiatrists use psychotherapy in its various forms for almost all conditions and diagnoses. Thus, a situation exists which differs considerably from the rest of medicine; that is, for the vast majority of psychiatric diagnoses there is only one basic treatment, psychotherapy. It would be excellent if this treatment was always effective, but it is not. The treatment is nonspecific, in some cases it is not effective and it depends, to a far greater degree than in medicine, upon the personality, the ego strength, and the competence of the therapist.

Acceptance of Treatment

In medicine the patient usually accepts medical treatment once he realizes he is ill. People with tuberculosis, heart disease, syphilis, and diabetes are constantly being discovered by medical surveys such as chest X rays, urinalyses, premarital and pre-employment examinations. Few people resist treatment when these undiscovered conditions are detected. Occasionally, the newspapers publicize a person of a certain religious faith who refuses medical treatment for himself or a member of his family and thus permits serious consequences to result. Such action causes anger and resentment in the general population. Editorials asking for laws to restrict this kind of behavior are not unusual, for it is generally accepted that if you are sick, you should receive medical treatment.

The psychiatrist's task would be easier if the same situation applied to mental illness. It does not, for at least three reasons: (1) exclusive of shock treatment for depression, there is no specific psychiatric treatment; (2) psychiatrists are not as widely available as are medical doctors; (3) there is a social stigma attached to psychiatric treatment. People who are able to recognize that they have defective egos often are reluctant to seek help because they feel the great prejudice which exists in many groups against the man who goes to a psychiatrist.

There are also many people, probably millions in this country, suffering from serious ego defects who do not realize it. Under present conditions these people will never get help. Nowhere have we approached the complicated task of beginning to screen them out and make them aware that they have defective egos. We have not the barest psychiatric measure which might be analogous to a chest X ray, a urinalysis, or a blood test. That is, we have no psychiatric screening device by means of which these people can recognize and appreciate their own illness, much as a man can appreciate his need for treatment when informed he has sugar in his urine. We are doing very little to solve this problem, an important part of mental hygiene. It is true that psychiatry seems to have its hands full with those who are seeking help and with those whom we have institutionalized for help, but we should not ignore this large group.

In addition to the fact that many mentally ill people will never receive treatment because they do not recognize their need for it, psychiatrists face another problem which is rare in medicine. Psychiatrists are called upon to give treatment to many people who do not want it, don't understand that they need it, and/or won't accept it. Nevertheless, when society recognizes that they are suffering from a defective ego, they may be legally committed to an institution for the purpose of improving their ego function. In medicine this almost never happens, except in the case of people suffering from Hansen's disease or leprosy.

Even though a treatment is available, nonspecific as it is, there is the problem of getting the patient to accept it because, unlike some medical treatment, in psychiatry the patient consciously or unconsciously must become actively involved or the treatment cannot be effective. Syphilis, for example, can be cured with an injection of several million units of penicillin; there are, however, no psychiatric drugs which will render a defective ego effective. There are some drugs which either help the ego to return to a previously more effective level or anesthetize the ego from uncomfortable feelings, thus allowing better functioning. Even forcefully administered shock treatments help in certain conditions, but experience shows that they are much more effective with a cooperative patient. The fact that administered treatments can never raise the level of ego functioning above a previous maximum is their great shortcoming.

Prolonged and nonspecific as it is at present, psychotherapy is the only treatment which can improve the level of ego functioning and thus make the ego more resistant to future defective functioning. Psychiatrists, therefore, must face the problem of the reluctance of some patients to accept treatment, and take the responsibility in many cases of treating patients who consciously as well as unconsciously resist treatment.

In general the principal psychiatric treatment is psychotherapy. All people with defective egos theoretically would benefit from psychotherapy. In practice, however, people with certain types of ego functioning make up the majority of the patients who receive psychotherapy. These include first, the anxiety neurotics and the symptom neurotics. These two groups almost always accept psychotherapy, either realizing themselves that they need psychiatric treatment or reaching that conclusion after their difficulty has been pointed out to them by others. For these people the general principles of psychotherapy apply exactly as they will be discussed.

In the large group which comprise the character neurotics and the sexual neurotics, the general principles of psychotherapy also apply. The only modification is that usually in these cases the patients come with very limited self-motivation, usually doing so at the insistence of the law or a member of the family. These patients try to manipulate the psychiatrist into refusing them treatment. They do so because psychotherapy causes them great anxiety for, in the relationship with the psychiatrist, they must face problems of getting along with the world that they desperately wish to avoid. Standing fast, the psychiatrist must not be tempted to respond to their desire by refusing them treatment. Although these neurotics have been thrown out of many helpful situations in the past, here they must be accepted and allowed to stay. In sexual neuroses the psychiatrist is the person through whom the patient can gain his sexual identity. These patients do everything possible to try to confuse the psychiatrist in his role, but again the psychiatrist must be firm.

When people with mildly psychotic ego structure come for help, psychotherapy needs to be slightly modified. In these cases the psychiatrist must be warm and accepting of everything the patient says except that which is crazy. He must not accept their psychoses. It is hoped that the psychosis will become alien to the patient as he regains contact with the world through the relationship with the psychiatrist. This relationship with a psychotic person is difficult to achieve and difficult to maintain. Often the psychotic patient is able to contact reality only in his relationship with the psychiatrist. In a sense he borrows a part of the psychiatrist's ego for his own as long as therapy continues. If the psychiatrist then withdraws, the patient often slips back into his psychosis—reality leaves with the withdrawal of the psychiatrist. Thus in many cases therapy must be continued long after the patient seems well.

The moderately depressed person who comes for psychotherapy should receive slightly different treatment from the aforementioned anxiety and symptom neurotics. He must be treated with less kindness and more matter-of-factly than most patients. It is hoped he may resent the psychiatrist's attitude and become angry at him. If he does so the anger which has been turned in against his own ego may be turned out against this accepting person who does not retaliate. As the anger comes out the depression lifts. If this is achieved, psychotherapy should proceed to strengthen the patient so depression is less likely to recur. Although stated simply here, psychotherapy with depressed patients is very difficult.

People with psychosomatic disease are almost always seen by psychiatrists only when they are referred by their physicians. Rarely will they avail themselves of psychiatric treatment on their own initiative. When they are well enough to come to the office the general principles of psychotherapy apply except that the psychiatrist, aware of their serious medical condition, must work in close harmony with the referring medical doctor.

Finally, a word about the treatment of children with defective egos, a large group who need psychotherapy but who are very difficult to treat in the ordinary way. In the case of very young children, ranging in age from two to six years, probably the best treatment is to place them in a good nursery school where they receive individual attention from teachers who are familiar with psychiatric problems of this age group. At the same time, their parents should receive psychiatric help to strengthen their egos in areas which relate to the child. If both parents are willing to cooperate, much can be accomplished to make the situation in the family more conducive to promoting ego growth in the child.

As the child grows older, from ages six to fourteen years, the problem may be handled in a different way. In these cases it is usually beneficial to have the child receive treatment from a skilled child therapist. This treatment embodies all the general principles of psychotherapy modified slightly because of the child's age. The parents should receive concurrent treatment.

In children fourteen years old or over, it is not always advisable to treat the parents. Although this decision is a matter of judgment, the inadequate parent-child relationship may be of such long duration that the parents' hostility to undergoing treatment might be communicated to the child and be an extra handicap in his treatment. Also, there are often influences on the child more important than those of the parent. If the parents want treatment for their own problems, that is excellent, but the child should be treated independently. He should be aware of the fact that his treatment is independent of his parents, and he should be helped to improve his ego in relationship to his parents without depending on them to change. As he improves, they often do change, but he should understand that his improvement is his own independent endeavor. He must receive the impression that he is being treated as an adult rather than as a child who cannot get along with his parents.

Treating the child independently serves to reduce the severe guilt feelings of both the child and the parent since, in these older children, each feels guilty over his part in the relationship. When only the child is treated, he feels less guilty because his parents are not involved, and the parents feel that they are not so much at fault. Because these children often have many problems in getting free of the parental relationship, the treatment is also important preparation for the child's independence.

The above groups, then, complete the list of those who might be seen in a private office or in an out-patient clinic. If they come at all, they accept treatment in some sense, and in all cases, except for the stated modifications, the general principles of psychotherapy apply. The vast majority of people with mild psychoses, depressions, character disorders, character neuroses, sexual neuroses, and psychosomatic diseases never voluntarily go to a psychiatrist. Many in this large group, which includes those with the most seriously defective ego functioning, are eventually institutionalized in our society. Institutional treatment of these patients is discussed separately in Chapter 22 after the chapter on psychotherapy.

21

Psychotherapy

PSYCHOTHERAPY MAY BE DEFINED AS ANYTHING, EXCLUSIVE of physical and drug therapies, a psychiatrist does which helps make ego functioning more effective. It must not be inferred that only psychiatrists can make ego functioning more effective, for this is far from the truth. People with defective egos are constantly getting help toward more effective ego functioning from many individuals besides psychiatrists. Psychiatrists can handle, directly in therapy or indirectly as in most institutional work, only the most seriously defective egos. Psychotherapy is not only a tool of specialized, psychiatrically trained people, but also something all people take part in at times, some knowingly, though most inadvertently.

If psychotherapy is not a specific psychiatric entity, what is it? The question is hard to answer in a concrete sense, but *whatever psychotherapy is, it is always the same thing.* By this I mean that whatever the process which goes on between people in which the ego functioning of one or more is made more effective, it is one, and only one, process. Whether it takes place between a schoolteacher and a pupil, a hospital aide and his psychotic patient, a psychiatrist and a phobic patient, or between any two (or more) people in any situation, psychotherapy is always the same. This thought leads to the following definition: *Psychotherapy is a meaningful, two-way relationship between two or more people in which a person whose ego is defective receives ego strength through the relationship with the person whose ego is more effective.* As children receive ego strength from good relationships with parents, so patients receive ego strength in the relationship with the psychotherapist.

The psychotherapist specializes and makes a career of this process and in so doing becomes a skillful and efficient practitioner. He then is able to apply his skill to the treatment of people with extremely defective egos who have been unable to get ego strength in any other way. The psychotherapist is qualified by his training to know a great deal about what is going on inside the patient and inside himself as the process proceeds. In an unclear situation he proceeds purposefully. Again, however, it must be stressed that with all the therapist's skill, *the ego strengthening which his patient achieves is in no way different or unique because it was achieved through therapy.*

An analogous situation involves a person who has a defective auto engine. He may work long and laboriously to fix it. The tools he uses and the techniques he employs might make a first-class mechanic shudder, but if he gets the job done, what he *actually did* which fixed the car is the same as the finest mechanic would have done. One way in which the situation is not analogous is that when *people* form a relationship in which one helps the other, it may be done inadvertently and as a by-product of the relationship. Between these people the process of psychotherapy proceeds at an unconscious level. Furthermore, in this relationship both may receive help toward more effective ego functioning, for, each being strong in different areas, they may give each other strength. This mutual improvement is the most common result of any good relationship between comparable people.

If the same people form a relationship specifically to help one or the other, the attempt may fail dismally because the skill is not there, the conscious effort to help spoiling the process. Although this statement does not mean that only psychiatrists can knowingly do psychotherapy, it does imply that, to do so purposefully, some extensive training is necessary. The end result of purposeful psychotherapy is not necessarily better than that due to inadvertent therapy, for all therapy must be judged by the same criterion—whether or not ego strengthening took place. Therefore, if one receives the strength from another to help him develop better ways of ego functioning, it makes no difference whether it is done purposefully or not. Finally, even in purposeful therapy with a psychiatrist, what takes place that is actually ego strengthening is not always immediately conscious to the patient; sometimes it is never conscious to him.

The purpose of this chapter is not to make a psychotherapist out of the reader, but rather to give some understanding into what, for many, is a mysterious process. There are certain definite factors basic to the process called psychotherapy when it is purposefully done between a therapist and a patient. There must be a warm, human, intimate relationship between the psychiatrist and the patient. The patient must perceive that the therapist is a person whom he can trust, who wants to help the patient for his own sake, and who will not desert him when he unburdens his difficulties. The patient must understand that the therapist is not afraid of becoming close and involved in this relationship, but that under no circumstances will the therapist take advantage of his position or of the vulnerable position of the patient. Realizing that the therapist is worldly enough to understand his problems and that he is actually interested in the struggles within the patient's ego, the patient must feel that real communication is possible so that he need not hide behind the walls of the pathological ego defenses which have served him so poorly in the past. Furthermore, he must have confidence in the ego strength of the therapist so that he can gain the potential strength which is in some way available to him from the therapist.

The process in which the patient learns how to use the ego strength which the therapist makes available to him in their relationship is the crux of psychotherapy. This process takes time. The patient gains strength from the therapist until it becomes his and he is able to use it as his own. As he does so, he suffers less because the general functions of the ego are markedly improved. The patient has the difficult, often painful, task of learning how best to use the relationship. Except in certain cases of psychosis or depression there is little the therapist can do to directly help him. Where there is ego weakness, as in the neurotic ego defects, attempts by the therapist to hurry the process usually have the opposite effect. During the long process the patient often becomes confused and discouraged. Feeling helpless and lost as the miraculous cure which he hoped for fails to materialize, he often blames the therapist, using all his old and unsuccessful ego defenses in an attempt to change the therapist. The therapist, firm and consistent, resists this pressure, so that it is the patient who must begin to change.

As he gains ego strength, the patient develops the ability to use his ego in better and more effective ways. As an additional part of the answer to the question of what psychotherapy is, a concept previously implied must now be stated. Psychotherapy always involves new experiences for the patient. This is in fact a prime requisite for psychotherapy because, if in his relationship with the therapist he experiences only old feelings, old fears, and old ways of thinking and acting, there can be no ego growth. Although the patient fears the new experiences, distrusts them, and runs from them, he experiences them. The therapist does not lecture, exhort, or direct him; nor does he fear the patient, misguide him, show anger toward him, laugh at him, or judge him. Warm and friendly, never hostile, he does not show emotions in the relationship which the patient won't understand.

Because ideally the therapist does little that the person has experienced before, the entire relationship is a new experience in which the patient's old and poor defenses do not work and in fact are not even necessary. In the new relationship the patient is free to let his ego grow in the absence of pathological defenses. Consistent in his relationship, the therapist does not react in many different ways. In his treatment of the patient he consistently shows kindness and strength so that their relationship has a solid base on which to grow. The patient's ego can never develop more effective functioning in an inconsistent relationship.

Finally, the therapist explains three relationships to the patient in a consistent, objective manner: (1) what is going on between the patient and the therapist; (2) what is going on between the patient and his needs; and (3) what is going on between the patient and the world. He makes the patient aware of how he is really functioning in these three areas. To do this a therapist has developed a skill that an untrained person does not have. The ability to point out these three relationships, and do it at the right time, is one of the major attributes of a good therapist. The patient's ego develops strength in the relationship, and the therapist must judge how much strength the patient's ego has gained. He must make these three areas clear to the patient only when he feels that the patient has developed enough strength to cope with them in a better way than he has coped with them in the past.

This, then, briefly describes good psychotherapy. Of course, it is much more complex in actual working than this short description implies; however, it is not the purpose of this discussion to explain complexities that are of primary concern only to a therapist. There are, however, certain popular misconceptions about psychotherapy which should be briefly explained, for they impede the understanding of many people.

Common Misconceptions

The most common misconception in all psychotherapy is the often fixed idea that therapy consists of the psychiatrist giving insight to the patient. People come to psychiatrists not understanding that it is a defective ego which has made therapy necessary, but rather with the idea that if they knew *why* they were feeling or acting as they did they would be comfortable. In no other branch of therapeutics, whether medicine, auto repairing, or animal disease, is such a "miracle cure" expected, yet the idea remains steadfastly fixed in peoples' minds about psychiatry and psychotherapy. Here, for reasons perpetuated both by psychiatrists and by many who write about psychiatry, this false idea has come to be almost gospel.

Just finding out what was wrong and how it happened, or even learning what is wrong now, cannot initiate more effective ego functioning. If one has an effective ego, this knowledge may be of great help because in that case the person has the ego to deal with the situation. If not, insight into the defective ego functioning does not help any more than does the understanding that Sam can't walk because he has a broken leg. This information is good to know, but much correct therapy is needed before Sam can walk. To find out that you are frightened of high places because certain important events happened in relation to important people early in your life does not help you get over the fear. Unless the ego is made more effective the phobia will continue unabated.

Movies, plays, and books often have a wonderful, exciting ending where the victim of a psychological catastrophe finds out the antecedents of his fear and becomes miraculously cured. Unfortunately, this pleasant sequence of events is always a figment of wishful thinking by the fiction writer, for in life it never occurs. Insight is valuable, probably the most valuable, knowledge a person can have if he can use it advantageously. Unfortunately, if one does not have an effective ego this same insight is worthless. It is because of this important difference that I stressed that the therapist must use his trained judgment to decide when to help patients toward insight.

If insight is obtained too early during therapy, or if it is given by well-meaning, psychiatrically oriented friends, it may even interfere with the process of ego growth. It does so because the patient grasps the insight to protect himself from advancing further in therapy. He rationalizes that he has received help, although what he really has gained is only another intellectual or word defense. A character familiar to many people is the one who, having had vast amounts of various psychotherapy, changed for the worse in the opinion of everyone except himself. In these cases insight served to produce a further ego defect—the person no longer realizes that he still has a defective ego.

Again it must be stressed that (in the ideal case) psychotherapy is the process which goes on between therapist and patient in which the patient's ego grows in all ways toward a more effective functioning. As his judgment improves he is able to utilize knowledge about himself so that it will help him. This therapy is never merely obtaining insight without the long, hard course of ego growth through the processes discussed in the beginning of this chapter.

It must be further stated that dealing with the patient's history is not directly related to psychotherapy. What is important is what is happening now. Many patients and even some therapists are content to work for long periods in the easy area of history where it is comfortable to contemplate how the patient became the way he is. This recounting of the past serves to insulate the patient from the important details of the present where his defective ego is now functioning. The history is important only as it helps the therapist work with present problems. Long histories and detailed psychological tests are more of interest than of help to the patient. A good therapist, who neither needs nor refuses a detailed history, recognizes the insulating and evasive nature of gathering this information. Although it almost always comes out in the course of any long treatment, history need not be solicited, nor is it meaningful unless the past is directly related to the present.

Thus, many of the accepted axioms in psychiatry and psychotherapy need to be re-examined to see if these old and revered procedures really have anything to do with the process of helping the patient. The process of psychotherapy is difficult enough without clinging tenaciously to procedures which, though revered, may not stand up under objective scrutiny. We must keep in mind the basic fact which has been stressed so many times in this book: ego strength comes through a good relationship with another person who has more ego strength. If this person is a trained therapist he has certain methods he can use to accelerate the process. There is, however, no short cut or magic way. Psychotherapy is a long, difficult process, but when it succeeds the patient has rendered his ego permanently more effective. With this start he can develop an even more effective ego because he is now able to make additional good two-way relationships with other people.

Finally it must be stated that the psychiatrist does not help the patient solve problems, or make him happy, or cause his anxiety to disappear. All that any therapist can hope to do is to help the patient toward developing a more effective ego. The patient then has additional and more successful ways to cope with his needs and with the world. If he is in an unhappy reality situation, nothing further can be done; he may, however, have the ego strength to cope with the situation differently or to endure it better. All things change, even the world changes slowly, so that what may be an intolerable situation for a person with a defective ego may in time become a more tolerable situation for a person with a more effective ego.

22

Treatment of Patients Who Are in Institutions

PATIENTS WHO ARE IN INSTITUTIONS NEED A VERY SPECIALized form of psychotherapy to help them toward more effective egos. For the most part they neither realize that they have defective egos nor understand and accept psychiatric help. Nevertheless, they must be treated by the application of the principles of good psychotherapy to the whole institutional program. Each person who has contact with the pa tient, ward, or inmate must be trained in the particular way he can help the patient. In the institution there must be created a therapeutic atmosphere in which the patients live. Thus, whether or not a patient understands or accepts treatment, he cannot avoid it. Although the kind of therapeutic atmosphere created varies, depending upon the type of ego defect with which the institution deals, many of the general principles are the same. These principles always include an atmosphere made up of kindness, consistency of treatment, acceptance of the patient as a human being, and the maximum number of new experiences for the patient.

Institutional Treatment of Character Disorders

Juvenile and Adult Delinquents

Jane is a seventeen-year-old juvenile delinquent. Having been picked up by the police twenty-one times for various offenses ranging from truancy to shoplifting, prostitution, and moderate involvement with non-opium narcotics, she has been in various juvenile halls and has received batteries of psychological tests, interviews with social workers, and several psychiatric evaluations. She can read and write fairly well, though she is almost devoid of academic education. With the stereotyped attitudes of the hostile and uninformed with regard to head shrinkers, she states,

Yeah, I was brought into the room, shown a lot of screwy pictures and asked to make up stories. Then I saw another guy, a head shrinker, I guess. He just lit a pipe and stared at me. I was supposed to talk, I guess, but I didn't know what to say. He asked me about my family. Hell, I ain't got no family: my mother used to try and make me sleep with her boy friends, so I run away. My old man is in San Quentin doing a twenty years to life stretch and I never seen him. My sisters are in foster homes and my brother is in the Navy, but I never seen him in years. The head shrinker stared some more, wrote a few notes and then let me go. Does he think I'm nuts or something? Maybe I am nuts to do the things I do, but, honest, when I'm doing those things I never think about it. I just do it. I don't ever think about anything much. It's funny, even when I'm in bad trouble I don't feel a thing.

This girl is typical of the adolescent character disorder seen in an institution for delinquents. Some don't talk as much, some talk more, but few have any understanding of their need for psychiatric help. Although mildly hostile to the people who have locked them up, they have little real feeling about anything. They exhibit this pattern of behavior because they have shattered, fragmented egos. The job of the institution is to repair the gaps in their egos to the extent that they can make a socially acceptable adjustment when they leave the institution. Institutions for juveniles usually have six to twelve months to do this job; many of the wards, however, come back again and again.

Treatment of the character disorders must be done in institutions in almost all cases. If the family can pay, a few seek psychiatric help because of family insistence. They rarely stay in treatment, and treatment rarely succeeds because far more is needed than a few hours a week with a psychiatrist, no matter how skilled he may be.

These people need a total treatment situation in a good institution where they will be accepted as human beings with the same basic needs as anyone else. The role of the psychiatrist in these cases is rarely to treat directly, but rather to work with all the people in the institution who come into contact with the wards. Corrective institutions, unlike mental hospitals, are not administered by psychiatrists. In fact it is only relatively recently that they have begun to employ psychiatrists at all. At present in good corrective institutions, the psychiatrist and the superintendent plan together to make the whole institution a therapeutic setting in which each contact with each employee is aimed at furthering ego growth. Unless a therapeutic atmosphere is created, the institution is inefficiently spending the taxpayers' money by serving only as a custodial facility.

Juveniles with shattered egos must be treated by everyone

with *kindness and consistency.* The institutional stay must provide a new experience, a good relationship with a staff of effective, interested adults. Treated strictly but fairly, the wards must only rarely be allowed poorly controlled behavior. Only people with strong egos, who can take responsibility for themselves, can benefit from permissive treatment. These young people need strict but understandable discipline, tailored to fit each individual. The discipline must always, first, be fair for the individual and, second, fair for the group. The situation is analogous to that of a family in which children are being raised correctly. It differs in institutions, not in quality but only in quantity, for there are so many to be helped. It is the personal contacts with people with strong egos which help the wards. Individuals and small groups interrelating in various activities with the staff is what is important. Nothing should be done for expediency; the individual must always be considered.

The staff must do more than make themselves available to the wards; they must be active in promoting relationships. These children have gaps in their egos and thus do not have the basic ego structure to make the necessary contacts. Thrusting himself into contact with them, the staff member must become involved and put the relationship on a personal basis. This is not office psychotherapy, it is much more active. The ward must feel the contact with the ego of the staff member because only then will part of it "rub off" and help fill the gaps in his ego. Relating to people who neither fear him nor show anger toward him, and who, at the same time, are much different from any of his previous associations is a new experience for the ward patient. He will try to get the staff member to respond in the old ways that he is used to because he expects and thinks he (his shattered ego) can handle this kind of response. The attempt to provoke the accustomed response from the staff members is made both individually and collectively, because the inmates of any institution for delinquents almost always form an institutional society which works directly to counteract any acceptance of help from the staff.

The inmates have a "prison code" which is anti-therapeutic and which enforces sanctions against those who co-operate and try to get help. The only way to combat this attitude is by the therapeutic atmosphere. When the institution workers do not respond in the old way, the hostility begins to lessen; the boy begins to believe that he can be accepted. He begins to have an identity he can feel and he can understand, for it wins him love and trust instead of fear and anger. As he discovers acceptance everywhere in a good institution, he begins to develop a sense of judgment and a sense of time. He uses his aggressiveness for his own social and intellectual gain, separating himself from the anti-therapeutic institutional society. When he makes such a break, it is certain that his ego has undergone considerable growth and that the institutional goal has been largely achieved.

The influx of younger and better trained people into institutional jobs is aiding progress toward the goal of ego growth. The punitive wall set up by some of the old-timers in the field is rapidly disappearing. More psychiatrists, psychologists, and social workers are now in the field, bringing with them knowledge of psychotherapy. Unfortunately, working against the creation of a therapeutic atmosphere is the increasing tendency for institutions for delinquents to grow in size, for with this growth it is difficult for the staff to maintain the all-important personal contacts. Also, the influx of psychiatric help often brings on an institutional dichotomy between the custodial staff and those who treat. This division is wrong and must not occur. Either everyone treats and a total therapeutic atmosphere exists, or the goal of filling the gaps in the ego will not be achieved.

In an institution with a strong therapeutic atmosphere much can be accomplished in a short time. Difficult as treatment seems to be with these boys and girls, they make rapid progress in a good setting. They must stay long enough for some ego growth to take place, yet not so long that the effect of custody stops further ego growth. The length of stay is a matter of judgment, varying with the severity of the ego disorder and the atmosphere of the institution.

The therapeutic atmosphere is in itself the basic psychiatric treatment for character disorders. Individual psychiatric treatment starts either after the initial ego repair has been accomplished or during the process. Individual psychotherapy is of little value in an institution where a therapeutic atmosphere does not exist.

The previous discussion, centered on juveniles, also applies with some modification to adult character disorders. The older person with a character disorder is very difficult to treat. Although he is more stable because age and experience have completed his ego by filling in many of the gaps, the resultant ego is weak, approaching that of the character neurotic. With the closing of the gaps he feels more anxiety, but because he fears and hates anxiety, he develops bad character defenses to avoid it.

Thus a character disorder blends into a character neurosis. With this modification to his ego, the adult character disorder is more stable, less impulsive, and more reasonable than the juvenile. He has a greater attention span and a better sense of identity. The general therapeutic atmosphere is still an important part of treatment, but now, as character neurosis supersedes character disorder in the older delinquent, he is more amenable to group and individual psychotherapy. Because group therapy is more feasible, it is the best choice and should be used in all institutions dealing with character disorders and character neurotics seventeen years old or more. Below age seventeen, group therapy has less effect; the therapeutic atmosphere must initiate the therapeutic process. As the older delinquents grow in ego strength, they find that they can accept anxiety and deal with it in ways which are not antisocial.

Thus the achievement of a therapeutic atmosphere is the goal of any institution dealing with delinquents—juvenile or adult. It is being attained in many institutions for juveniles and also in some state and federal adult reformatories. The numbers of therapeutic institutions must continue to grow because money spent on custody alone is, for the most part, wasted money. Institutions should provide an opportunity for ego growth, for without it recidivism will continue at the present high rate.

Important as is the institutional therapeutic atmosphere, equally important are transition living quarters for those who have no home and for whom a foster home cannot be found. This living arrangement must also have a therapeutic atmosphere and must be attractive enough to be accepted by the released inmate. Augmenting the present parole system, the transition home is a necessary part of the rehabilitation of many adolescent and adult delinquents; an individual's ego can advance only so far even in a good institution. He usually needs further help in making the transition back to society.

Institutional Treatment of Sexual Neurotics

The sexual neurotics who are institutionalized for treatment are usually those persons who attack, seduce, or molest young children of either sex or who attack women. Also, often institutionalized are the homosexuals, Peeping Toms, men who dress in female clothes or who masquerade as females, and men who expose their genitalia in public. The varieties of sexual aberration are legion, yet, as previously explained, they are all character neurotics with inadequate sexual identity. Most of the sexual neurotics institutionalized are males, since females who exhibit these tendencies are rarely so feared that they are publicly prosecuted.

The institutional treatment of this particular group is not highly successful. It is difficult to help a person who has reached eighteen to twenty-five years of age without attaining moderate security in his sexual role. The usual good institutional treatment may help a little, although this help seems partly to stem from the fact that they are safe in the institution. Sexual neurotics get along well and cause no difficulty when they are segregated and removed from the social pressure of proving their identity. Group therapy is the most widely used form of psychotherapy; these patients, however, change very slowly. The most that can be expected at the present time is that a period of institutionalization may help differentiate among those of this group who are dangerous to society and those who are not. The ones who are judged to be dangerous must be kept segregated indefinitely in institutions. This is a difficult judgment to make, but when it is not made an innocent member of society may pay with his life.

INSTITUTIONAL TREATMENT OF HEROIN ADDICTS

At the present time there is no good treatment for heroin addicts; in fact one could frankly say that there is not even a poor treatment. As explained previously, the addict is a person with a severe character disorder who has found his own cure, albeit pathologically. The heroin acts, in a sense, to fill the gaps in his ego—it fills his needs, gives him an identity, and removes all the emptiness. From his standpoint he neither needs nor wants treatment. He wants only heroin in sufficient supply to support his habit.

When we attempt to treat a heroin addict we first cut off his supply of the drug. The holes or gaps in his ego are then opened wide, and he is left without any ability to function or to fill his needs. He is sharply and distressfully aware of his lack of identity and of his emptiness. Of all the empty people, the drug addict deprived of his drug is probably the most painfully empty. Looking at the withdrawal of the drug as cruel and unnecessary treatment, he does not have the ego strength to enable him to realize that it is done for his own good. From his viewpoint, when he is deprived of heroin and told he must accept institutional treatment, to him it is as if his hands were shackled behind his back while he is told that he will be well again if he can only wait until the heavy steel handcuffs rust off. Then he will have the use of his hands again and everything will be just fine.

This viewpoint puts the person who is attempting to treat him in a very difficult position because the addict goes much further than just not accepting treatment. He resists it for it causes him great suffering, and he knows that one simple injection will cure all his pain. Often he is not only deprived of his heroin but also locked up in jail or prison for long periods where no attempt is made at therapy to help close the ego gaps which, in a sense, we have recreated by our legal actions.

Since, in medical language, we are dealing with a disease which at present is 98 to 99 per cent fatal, it behooves us to look for some better treatment. There is nothing to lose and much to gain if the cure rate can be raised even to 10 per cent from its present level of less than 2 per cent. A group of addicts in Los Angeles are living in a (modified) communal society for the purpose of resisting the habit. They have banded together in an apartment as a sort of Narcotics Anonymous. Their response to the problem shows that some, at least, have enough judgment to recognize their predicament and try to help themselves.

Youths who have not been addicted very long can be helped if they receive long periods of treatment in institutions with a good therapeutic atmosphere where they are not mixed with too many older addicts. The latter create an anti-therapeutic attitude which makes the therapeutic task very difficult. Older addicts are almost incurable; the only course for them is lengthy confinement in a good institution. Perhaps we should even consider an addicts' prison colony, where they could live more normally than in institutions, but still be separated from society and from drugs. The prison colony concept, foreign to most Americans, is accepted in some countries. It works well in some criminal cases, though I know of no specific use for drug addicts.

Another possible solution to the problem of handling adult addicts is to make drugs available to registered addicts through state clinics. There is no good reason for not giving this oft-proposed idea a trial. The British claim that for them it works reasonably well. It certainly would cut out some of the criminal underpinnings of drug addiction. Perhaps it would work with selected addicts; a research program could be instituted to select them. Of the many arguments against state clinics, the principal ones are that it expresses a defeatist attitude and that it is a public toleration of vice. To attempt this solution offends that rapidly shrinking part of our egos which clings to puritan ideals; still, we tolerate much vice in our society. If a trial period led to a workable program, it would be a strong weapon against all the crime linked to drug addiction.

Institutional Treatment of Psychotic Patients

At the present time in the United States there are over 500,000 people institutionalized in mental hospitals. The vast majority of these people have egos so thick and rigid that they cannot live in society. Probably there is an equal number almost as sick who are not hospitalized for various reasons or who are waiting for hospital beds to be vacated. The recognition that psychosis was a mental illness which would respond to treatment rather than cruel confinement started in modern times with Pinel in France in 1792. Since that time awareness has increased so that it is now a generally accepted concept in psychiatry. Although there are many in our society who scoff at psychiatric treatment for delinquent behavior, who feel neurotic people just need a "kick in the pants," and who claim that there is no such thing as psychosomatic disease, most of them readily accept the idea of mental hospitals to treat the psychotic patient.

Accepted as this idea is, however, much improvement is required in the quality of the treatment which mental patients receive. From time to time newspapers and crusading journalists inform the people of the cruel truths about conditions in some public and private mental hospitals. The aroused public reacts—some gains are made—but then the furor subsides and the patients, though better off than before, still do not receive good treatment.

A prevalent idea is that psychiatrists do not know how to treat psychotic patients, that recovery is just a question of confinement and chance. This idea is incorrect—in this field psychiatrists know how to provide good treatment. The problem is that institutional psychiatrists rarely have the proper personnel and the adequate facilities required to give treatment which, in turn, will lead to recovery for well over 50 per cent of the admitted patients. Again, as in the treatment of delinquents, it is necessary to create a therapeutic atmosphere. It is not the same atmosphere as in the treatment of character disorders, however, because the ego structure of the psychotic patient is radically different, and he reacts differently.

The treatment of psychotic patients is easier than the treatment of character disorders, for they do not establish an anti-therapeutic society (prison code), which actively resists treatment. On the contrary, there is no organized society at all because their principle problem is that of withdrawal from the world into the world of their own egos. Therefore, the therapeutic society has an initial important goal of reducing the isolation of these patients. To accomplish this goal, the hospital staff members work with the part of the ego still in contact with the world and attempt to enlarge it. They act in a kind and accepting manner toward all patients except in the area of their psychosis, where they reject what the patient may do or say that is crazy. For example, when a patient says he is Jesus Christ, the staff accepts him only as Joe Smith, the man he really is. The hope is that if the staff, whom he knows and is beginning to trust, accept him as he is, he can give up the delusion of omnipotence. The transition is accomplished gradually. The many people who see each patient must all present the same firmly consistent attitude because, with the first sign of inconsistency, the patient becomes frightened and often withdraws into his psychosis. Much long and arduous work of winning a patient back to reality can be inadvertently undone in a few moments by someone who does not know the patient.

Although some aspects of mental illness are frightening, the people who work with these patients must not be frightened; fear in the atmosphere tends to perpetuate psychosis;

lack of fear tends to make psychosis unnecessary. The psychiatrist in the mental hospital must lead the way for the rest of the staff. He is the sole leader of the therapeutic community, contrary to the situation in corrective institutions where this responsibility is shared. When he has a staff who accept him as a leader, who discuss with him their feelings about their work and their patients (not themselves, this is not staff therapy) and who are genuinely motivated to help, psychotic patients get well. There is then little need for drugs, restraints, shock treatments, or wet packs. Because psychotic patients are rarely dangerous, the doors may be opened, doing away with the old idea of incarceration. Locking them up and preventing free social movement only serves to increase their feelings of isolation. Furthermore, in order to reduce isolation and increase staff and family contacts, hospitals must be made smaller and brought nearer to the cities where the patients live. It is easy to create a therapeutic atmosphere in an adequately staffed ward of thirty patients, but impossible in an understaffed ward of two hundred patients.

Patients should never be given up as incurable. Some doctors feel that if a man is psychotic for more than five years, the case is almost hopeless. This is not true. Good treatment often is as effective with patients who have been sick for years as with people who have just become psychotic. In many cases, a man who becomes psychotic does so after a great struggle within his ego, and it seems to take a while before his ego is ready for change. Psychosis is almost a rest for him after that struggle; thus we should not expect to help all the acutely psychotic immediately. Sometimes if immediate treatment fails, later treatment helps, although in a good hospital treatment is continual.

Finally, it must be recognized that, in contrast to character disorders, persons who become psychotic were in many cases skilled, well-functioning people in the community and that they have not necessarily lost their skills because they are psychotic. They should be encouraged to perform work around the hospital at as high a level as possible. They should never be asked to engage in silly or irrelevant activities. Many patients, still severely psychotic, have expressed their distaste of childish games, entertainment, and activities foisted off on them because they were "poor schizy patients." This attitude, bitterly resented, cannot help to break down their wall of isolation. Activities should be explained to the patients whether or not they seem to understand. We cannot know what goes on inside a man who has rejected reality, but we must treat him as though he could understand our treatment and activity program. A cardinal rule to follow is: Never underestimate the ability of the patient to understand the method and motivation of the therapist.

Along with the therapeutic atmosphere, individual psychotherapy and group therapy have their place in the treatment of psychotics. Psychotherapy is an excellent addition to any program, but creating and maintaining the therapeutic atmosphere is primary; formal psychotherapy comes next. In working with psychotics the role of the psychiatric staff and technicians is less active than in the treatment of the character disorders. It is more difficult to judge the best way to approach the psychotic patient. The staff must be able to motivate each patient selectively. A man can't be pushed out of psychosis, but the staff must sense when he is ready for active attention. When the patient makes his "move" it must be accepted, because patients do not often move toward reality. Thus it is important to hold frequent staff conferences in which each staff member gives his impressions of the patient including the level of the patient's receptivity toward returning to reality. Also, it is from these conferences that patients who are ready for institutional psychotherapy can be selected.

The relationship between the mental hospital and the community needs improvement. The Veterans' Administration and some states have instituted a foster-home plan wherein private families keep amenable chronic mental patients for long periods. This limited plan has been successful, helping many to progress further than they could have in the hospital. For discharged patients with no home, hospital-sponsored facilities, such as supervised residences where they can stay while they are becoming reintegrated into the community have proved helpful. Also needed are employment agencies especially for convalescent mental patients and facilities for family consultation with social workers, so that families can better understand the problem of the patients' return to the community.

Institutional Treatment of Depression

A small, but significant, proportion of patients in any mental hospital are diagnosed as depressed. There are other names for this condition, such as affective psychosis, depressed state, and involutional melancholia. The complaint and treatment, however, are the same whatever the name. The patients are sad, depressed, dejected, and immobilized. They may or may not be psychotic, or they may be psychotic at times. The general features of the psychosis, if it exists, are unrealistic self-depreciation, delusions, and wishes for death.

Many depressed patients, however, seem to be psychologically accessible to the therapist. Talking and relating well, they often seem to be amenable to psychotherapy. They may make some progress, seem to brighten, but then slip back into depression. This cycle can continue for long periods.

In many cases, the objective therapist notices that the patient is getting sicker and that he appears even worse around the therapist than around the regular hospital personnel. This situation might be explained by the type of ego defect which predominates in depression: the ego turns the anger reaction against itself. In some cases relating to the therapist is a burden to the patient's anger-immobilized ego because the better the relationship, the less the patient is able to express the anger causing the depression.

The best treatment for many depressed patients is electric shock therapy. Discussing the selection of who is to receive shock and how it is to be given is beyond the scope of this book. Shock, perhaps, acts as an ego-clearing mechanism similar to clearing a computing machine in preparation for another problem. As the anger is temporarily cleared from the system, releasing the ego from its anger-induced immobilization, the depressed patient usually perks up and feels better. The improvement is very often permanent if the situation causing the anger has been changed, though sometimes the remission continues even if there has been no obvious change. The lasting beneficial effect of shock treatment might be explained by reasoning that once anger gets into the ego of the depressed person, it can't get out—that is, the ego has no internal strength to remove it—but when anger has been cleared from the ego by an external agent, electric shock, it becomes active and flexible, able to perform its general functions satisfactorily again. Depression may not recur unless another severe loss takes place. It is considered good principle to treat the patient using psychotherapy for a time even after he says he feels fine. This period seems to help strengthen the ego so that it is less likely that depression will recur.

A constant danger in depressed patients is suicide. As discussed in Part II, depressed patients are apt to commit suicide, not at the height of their depression, but when they are feeling better; either after coming out of a severe depression or while still mobilized, prior to going into a depression. They must not be ignored when they talk of suicide because studies show that the person who talks of suicide is more likely to attempt it than is a person who never mentions this possibility.

Finally, depressed patients should be hospitalized for as short a period as possible. When they feel better they should leave the hospital and be advised to go back to work, for they can then constructively dissipate any residual anger by living and reacting with people. Inactivity compounds their problem and should be discouraged. They need the opposite of the hackneyed advice, "All you need is a good rest," because when they are inactive they are not resting. With their hope for psychological rest in activity, they need strong, directive handling to get them to resume working. The psychiatrist is often opposed by the family when he acts rashly to galvanize these patients into needed activity.

Institutional Treatment of Psychosomatic Diseases

The psychiatric treatment of a person suffering from severe psychosomatic disease can, at times, mean the difference between the life and death of the patient. In diseases such as asthma, ileitis, and colitis, and occasionally ulcers, death may occur despite the best medical care. Many competent medical doctors who have successfully treated these difficult diseases ascribe their success to their ability as psychotherapists. The strongest reason for psychiatrists to have a good medical training is for the treatment of these increasingly diagnosed conditions. From a psychiatric standpoint, however, many patients do not get the type of treatment considered best for their conditions. These patients need a combined medical-psychiatric approach, which by our present-day practice of medicine, means joint treatment by a psychiatrist and a medical doctor. For the treatment to work, however, it must be a truly cooperative effort.

Although he has a vital stake in the outcome of the treatment, the patient is not directly involved in one of its most important phases, the relationship between the psychiatrist and the medical doctor. If they do not have complete mutual trust and respect for the treatment skill which each brings to the case, and if they do not cooperate fully with each other, the patient suffers. A patient with a psychosomatic disease is often caught between two conflicting schools of therapy: that emphasizing the medical approach and that emphasizing the psychiatric approach. Many times he uses this conflict to undermine the relationship between his doctors in order to resist psychological help. Having adapted himself to his psychosomatic illness, he is frightened when confronted with its psychological causes because he fears they will cause him more pain. Also, consciously he fears that the medical help he feels he needs for the illness will be reduced if he admits to himself that it has any psychological basis.

If the two doctors cannot cooperate as described above, it is better for the patient if one or the other takes over complete charge of the case. Assuming cooperation between the doctors, they must communicate to the patient that a large part of his treatment is psychological. At the same time, both doctors must reassure the patient that they understand the organic disease and will alleviate it with all the medicines and medical skills available. While doing so, however, they never vary from their basic psychological approach. The patient may insist on his incapacity, as did one asthmatic patient who said, "Jeez, Doc, I can't even breathe, much less talk; what do you want from me?" He talked, though, and breathed better, gaining considerable relief from his serious, medically resistant asthmatic condition.

The psychiatric treatment in the hospital is basically individual psychotherapy, as described in Chapter 21. The difference here is that the psychiatrist must visit frequently at the patient's bedside, often for long periods during acute and severe phases of the illness. Then as the patient recovers, the treatment may taper off in time and frequency of visits so that, when the patient leaves the hospital, regular out-patient psychotherapy can be instituted.

IV

MENTAL HYGIENE

Introduction

Mental hygiene is the broad application of sound psychiatric principles to a community in order to help more people develop effective egos. It should not be confused with psychiatric treatment, a very specific and limited application of the same principles. The objective of any program of mental hygiene is to increase the level of ego effectiveness of a whole community and thereby reduce significantly the number of people with defective egos.

To delineate a program of mental hygiene which can accomplish this goal it is necessary to examine closely the key portion of the definition of mental hygiene: "application of sound psychiatric principles." For explanation it may be divided into two major parts: application, and sound psychiatric principles. Application, the first part of the definition, may in turn be divided into two categories: method of application and instrument of application; or, in more simple terms: How can mental hygiene be implemented and who can do the implementing? First, let us examine the question of how it can be done, for answering that question involves a basic problem..

We all desire to function more effectively. We have learned that through application of sound psychiatric principles better functioning is possible and certainly, as described in the section on treatment, psychotherapy is an application of sound psychiatric principles. Does psychotherapy, however, apply to all people, whether or not their egos are defective? I will answer this much belabored question by stating that it does not. Many people in our society have the capacity to function much more effectively without psychotherapy. For them it would be a tedious and inefficient road to a more effective ego.

In contrast to people with defective egos, who need psychotherapy, people with *moderately effective ego function* can improve themselves without psychotherapy by learning sound psychiatric principles through direct and indirect education. Whereas psychotherapy is always indirect, education can be applied directly to a mental hygiene program. As long as their egos are not grossly defective, people can learn much about how they function and, by using this knowledge, can improve their performance. The more that effective people understand about how their egos operate, the more effectively they will function. The direct education can be in the form of a book such as this one, lectures, movies, or any other educational medium. For a mental hygiene program to reach its objective the direct education must be supplemented by indirect education using a trained person who can stimulate thought without formally teaching, a process to be discussed in detail later.

Next let us examine the people who can teach mental hygiene. The most important teacher is the individual parent, who, in applying to himself and his family the sound psychiatric principles he has learned, forms the backbone of any mental hygiene program. Through the activity of a vigorous mental hygiene agency, the community will have more parents with effective egos, who will raise a greater percentage of children with effective egos. The book has introduced in Part I a theoretical exposition of sound psychiatric principles. In the following chapter some of these principles are expanded and discussed under the heading of family mental hygiene.

Although some communities have mental hygiene programs, these are restricted to the treatment of the seriously mentally ill. This treatment agency will reduce somewhat the numbers of people with severely defective egos, but it can contribute little toward raising the over-all level of ego functioning in the community. Still needed is a working civic mental hygiene agency with no responsibility for the treatment of the mentally ill. Today no such agency exists anywhere in the United States. Though seemingly more pressing, the treatment of the mentally ill is no more important than the promotion of a community mental hygiene program. Because no such program is in effect anywhere, I will outline, following the chapter on family mental hygiene, the working of a mental hygiene agency which might be implemented by any community at moderate cost but with possible far-reaching benefit.

23

Family Mental Hygiene

EVERY PARENT DESIRES TO DEVELOP A METHOD OF CHILD rearing which will help his child attain effective ego functioning—that is, a firm sense of identity, good judgment, and a forceful, aggressive ego. In the first part of this book it was pointed out that initially the child must learn to develop two-way relationships with his mother and those about him. From these relationships, assuming they are with people who have moderately effective egos, his own ego develops effectively. In this chapter the process is examined more closely.

Let us again look at a child who arrives home a few days after birth. As previously explained he has the same needs as everyone else, and he has these needs throughout his life. Continually struggling to stay alive and to gain satisfactions, he desires pleasure and withdraws from pain. At birth he has his full physical and mental potential which, barring great physical misfortune, will not change. What he does not have at birth are the methods to develop his physical and mental potentialities. The more successfully he develops them, the more effective human being he will be.

The newborn babe has the capacity both to benefit himself and others and to do great harm to our society and to himself. When Adolf Hitler and Abraham Lincoln were small infants looking through blurred eyes at their new surroundings, both with vast potential, no one could have forseen their futures. Though it is not apparent at his birth, a newborn human has within him great power due to his great potential. If we see a loaded dynamite truck rolling down the highway, we exercise much caution and hope that the driver will do the same, for we recognize instantly that he is entrusted with the care of tremendous destructive force. When the parents and neighbors of Adolf Hitler looked at him in his perambulator, they did not see the thousands of truckloads of dynamite within that tiny babe. Nor did they know that due to him many millions of people, including some of these very neighbors, were to perish in later years. Thus, under any social system, in any part of the world, rich or poor, educated or illiterate, the newborn babe is an unknown with enormous potential power.

It follows, therefore, that the first principle of family mental hygiene is *parental responsibility*, the conscientious responsibility to the child and to society to guide this powerful potential with care. From it, responsibility develops in the child; without it, learning responsibility becomes haphazard. Caring for the physical needs of the child and giving him love and affection are only a part of parental responsibility. In addition, the parent should provide an environment in which the child can establish his identity, learn good judgment, and develop a forcefully functioning ego that can serve him well in later life.

Parental Responsibility

The most important part of correct child raising is the parent's assumption of responsibility for his role. Comfortable or uncomfortable, a parent must be prepared for a long, exhausting, and not necessarily happy undertaking, for there is no built-in assurance that raising a child will be rewarding. The sacrifices of parenthood, the joys of raising children are glib phrases, easily mouthed, but unfortunately without meaning to many people who derive little more than physical and psychological misery from the fulfillment of their biologic role. They, in turn, bring forth a group who repeat the unhappy cycle; they make it unhappy because they do not have the ego strength to assume the responsibility required for their role. In fact, they do not know what their role really is—they have no identity as parents. For these people family mental hygiene is, unfortunately, only an empty phrase. For their children the mental hygiene which leads to an effective ego is obtained outside the home or not at all.

Most people, however, do have a basic sense of marital and parental responsibility. Although they are willing to suffer and sacrifice moderately for the pleasures of bringing new lives into the world, they are unsure of what to do when the children actually arrive. For these parents a discussion of sound psychiatric principles can be extremely helpful. They want to be told something about raising a child and they look to experts. One expert, Dr. Benjamin Spock,[1] has written one of the most widely read books in the English language. Although much of what he writes is under the heading of physical child care, he has developed a psychologically sound point of view in which all his physical advice is carefully framed. He has attempted to help parents by taking some of the responsibility for their child's welfare. Parents depend on his book because what he says makes sense, and it works; however, in the area of ego growth, even the best books can only provide a discussion of general principles. The parent who wishes to raise his child with an effective ego must accept one basic fact: He must do most of the job himself—he can't depend on books, articles, or experts.

Although books can teach a parent the basic principles of ego functioning, they can never tell him what to do in a specific psychological situation. Raising a child is, of course, a long series of specific psychological situations. When the child has a temper tantrum, it is up to the parent to handle it then and there. He must handle it so that it benefits the child and relieves his tension. Books and experts are confus-

[1] Benjamin Spock: *Baby and Child Care*, New York: Pocket Books, Inc., 1946.

ing in these situations; they rarely agree, and, in any case, the experts who write them cannot know the fact of the specific situation.

To clarify the point under discussion, which can't be stressed too strongly: *Almost anything the parent does is right if he is willing to take responsibility for his actions relating to the child.* This statement can be explained by continuing the example of the temper tantrum. Here the child has exploded emotionally because of some frustration. He has exploded to his parent because his parent, responsible for everything in the child's eyes, must be responsible for this frustration. This responsibility is always clear in the eyes of the child; he endows his parent with it whether or not the parent wants to take it. The parent can follow any of several courses depending upon how willing he is to acquiesce in the child's thinking. Suppose that the child is having a tantrum because he has carelessly broken a beloved toy. Whose responsibility is this? The parent can take it all by running to buy a new toy, or he can take none of it by ignoring the tantrum. Although in either case the tantrum stops, we must ask: How is the child affected? In one case he succeeds in placing complete responsibility for his frustration on his parent, thus avoiding it himself. In the other case, he begins to learn that his parent, omnipotent as he may seem, will not take responsibility for something which is rightfully the child's responsibility. Obviously in this case the latter course is preferable.

However, it is still necessary to clarify the statement that *any course the parent follows is correct providing he takes responsibility for his actions.* That is, he takes *responsibility for his own actions completely*, but for only that part of the *child's* responsibility which is logical in the situation. Thus a parent who ignores a tantrum in his three-year-old-child precipitated by his ripping his play panda is acting correctly because the parent is *not* taking responsibility for the accident. The same parent who ignores a three-year-old crying because he has broken a fragile, complicated toy would be acting wrongly toward the child, because he would be avoiding responsibility rightfully his, namely, allowing the child to play with a toy requiring maturity beyond his age level.

Similar reasoning can be expanded in many directions. The father who buys his sixteen-year-old a car must take part of the responsibility for lower grades in school. He can't point to the boy's promises to keep up his grades because relying on these promises is not logical in this situation. The same father who, refusing his son a car, must cope with the succeeding fireworks, is taking responsibility for the situation —enduring the pain— but perhaps happily sharing the scholastic success following his decision. Many more examples could be added, all showing the same principle: The parent assumes responsibility, even at the cost of pain, for that part of the child's welfare that is logically his. His share of the responsibility for the child's actions diminishes as the child grows and begins to take responsibility for his own actions, which he must do if the parent plays his role correctly.

The discerning reader may feel that the statement that the parent take only the responsibility logical to the situation was skipped over too quickly. How does the parent know what is logical and what is not? Although no one can tell you exactly what your responsibility is, sometimes outside sources can offer valuable guidance to help make this always-difficult decision. For example, a daily newspaper in Los Angeles published a study which showed that after a teen-age boy gets a car his grades drop two levels. If he has been only an average student, he may well not finish school. If someone shows the results of this study to a parent, it should be good ammunition for him to decide to defer buying his high school boy a car.

Most parents have the necessary judgment. They are reluctant, however, to assume the proper responsibility. When they do, it is more likely that their children will grow up with highly effective egos. When parents vacillate, shift in their assumption of responsibility, run to others for help, join groups for protection, and abrogate their individual judgment to some "expert" advice, they will contribute little to an effective ego in their children. The parent, suffering a little pain, even making a few mistakes in rearing his child, if he does so honestly and on his own, well fulfills many of the requirements of family mental hygiene. It cannot be concluded, however, from the above discussion that parents who do not accept their proper responsibility necessarily raise children with defective egos. But their children will need to find the stimulus for ego growth elsewhere, making it a less sure, less satisfactory process.

Parental Direction

There is one main reason for the uncertainty concerning the part direction plays in parental responsibility. That reason is the heritage of the misguided group who promulgated "progressive" or permissive child raising; a method of raising children with minimal parental guidance and discipline. In opposition to the teaching of this group, the correct use of parental direction is simple and logical. It follows the course of the parent assuming total responsibility for directing the child's activities at birth to his relinquishing direction completely when the child reaches adulthood.

As the child grows older, as his ego matures, he is better able to direct his own activities, or, in another sense, he takes more responsibility for himself. Under the progressive or permissive system the small child is allowed to direct his own activities—to engage in his own fanciful pursuits with no parental interference. The rationale is that parental direction warps the child's ego growth through frustration, and that frustration is undesirable because it inhibits a child from developing his true potential.

However, the child left without guidance is confused and dismayed. Feeling abandoned and unloved by parents who do not direct him in activities in which he is still too immature to direct himself, the child regards the permissive parent not as a benefactor but rather as a person who doesn't care. His tantrums, therefore, are directed not at any frustration but at his parents from whom he is desperately asking guidance. Unfortunately, parents who raise their children without direction can escape the results for awhile, because young children have little power to do harm. When later, for example, daughter becomes sexually promiscuous, they attempt direction, but it fails. It fails because during adolescence the controls developed in childhood through proper direction must take over. If direction was lacking, controls are poorly developed. These parents see their responsibility when the child is capable of doing harm to himself or others, but it is often too late: To inculcate inner controls in an older child is at best difficult, and sometimes impossible.

In school also early direction and discipline must be firm so that they may be safely relaxed as the child progresses up the educational ladder. Having learned the basic scholastic skills, he can now proceed on his own. If there is a general criticism of education in America which I can make, it is that there is too much direction at the college level and too little in the preparatory years. College students are adults, but few colleges treat them as such. Thus a true liberal education where the professor stimulates his thinking, adult students and shares his knowledge with them is difficult to obtain in this country.

Parental Emotions

A final important part of parental responsibility is the parent's emotions as they affect the child. Much has been written about how parents should try to control their emotions, to substitute reason for anger, and to present a calm, collected, unemotional atmosphere for the child. It is important, however, that this control does not stifle parental emotions. Fortunately, most parents are blessed with the kind of children who easily inspire adequate parental emotions. As a child grows, he develops emotions by experiencing emotional reactions from those around him. The parent who is able to give reasonable vent to his emotions provides an honest emotional atmosphere, one where, by the nature and degree of parental response, the child can quickly learn when his parents are pleased or displeased. Although in an atmosphere where emotions are freely expressed a child may be buffeted, at least he is not puzzled.

A parent who carefully and calmly notes his child's behavior, later to discipline him, confuses the child. Punishment of the child should never be cold or calculating, but should be quick and accompanied by anger. Bertrand Russell[2] wisely said, "Never strike a child except in anger." If you are angry, one or two good whacks to discharge the angry emotions and let the child feel that he has at least gained peace at the expense of his pain is good discipline. Formal, corporal discipline is cold and puzzling because the child does not learn from it. The value of good punishment is the release of emotional tension so that the transgression becomes less charged with feeling. The air is cleared.

The child raised in an atmosphere of permissiveness where transgressions are overlooked goes to desperate ends to provoke an emotional response from his parents. When it does come, often so much tension has been built up that the child is frightened and overwhelmed at the outburst from his usually controlled parents. He then fears his parents and wonders what they may do next. Under these circumstances he is not prepared by the beneficial effect of continuous spontaneous emotions and his responses may be stunted.

As explained in Part I, emotions are the rewards as well as the punishment built into the ego operation. In an atmosphere where emotions are out in the open, they can amply reward the individual. When emotions are covered up too long, they may break out uncontrolled or they may fester within, causing depression or psychosomatic disease. If they

---

[2] I read this statement several years ago in a book by Bertrand Russell; now I cannot locate the book. The statement is so apt that I feel I have to quote it even without being able to locate the exact source.

are constantly released before tension builds too high, the child learns to develop many good ways to discharge his emotions and to experience their rewards. Children who grow up in an atmosphere of love, acceptance, responsibility, discipline, direction, and freely vented emotions have an excellent chance to develop strong, flexible egos, and to acquire a firm identity of themselves as valued human beings.

24

Community Mental Hygiene

COMMUNITY MENTAL HYGIENE IS THE APPLICATION OF SOUND psychiatric principles to a community to raise the general level of ego functioning in that community. I know of no community where an organized agency performs this function today. Again it must be stressed that mental hygiene is not the job of present community clinics and social agencies, because they are established for people with defective egos. In order to emphasize the distinction, this agency should be separate from the treatment agencies.

The purpose of this agency is to teach psychiatrically sound principles to individuals and organizations in the community using a group program. Ideally, the people who work in the agency should have broad psychiatric training in community mental hygiene, training not yet available specifically, although many psychiatrists have enough experience to do the work. Experience with the mentally ill is valuable, but equally valuable is group experience with mentally healthy people.

Assuming that a psychiatrist with wide experience is appointed mental hygiene director, what should he and could he do to successfully apply good psychiatric principles to the community? Probably first he would make his department known in the community. A little publicity, augmented by a series of lectures on mental hygiene to various groups, would begin the education of the community. His initial audiences might include schools, churches, boys' and girls' organizations, service clubs, women's clubs, business groups, professional groups, and unions. His agency would also address governmental groups and agencies not directly connected with the mentally ill, such as the police and health and welfare departments.

Mental hygiene must be sold through education; if it is done poorly, later setbacks will jeopardize the program.

Services of a Mental Hygiene Agency

The primary service of a mental hygiene agency would be to make available people, well grounded in psychiatrically sound principles, to groups in the community who have problems in interpersonal relations. Suppose the Boy Scouts apply to the agency to help train scoutmasters. The agency would provide personnel to organize and administer a workshop consisting of a series of sessions for these leaders. The sessions would be divided into two main parts, the direct education and the indirect education. In direct education the leader would present some material on ego function, reactions or defenses. A variety of ways to present the information is possible—lecture, movie, slides, or perhaps a psychological discussion of popular literature, plays or movies. With any method the leader would always strive to make the material living and understandable to the group. Simple material would be presented first, later working into more complex presentations.

The indirect education would be less formal with either large or small discussion groups. Subjects could be introduced using the didactic material as a starting point, or the leader could encourage free discussion within the group. Depending upon the caliber of the group, the leader might hold the initial sessions to more general principles. Later as the group becomes more comfortable he could encourage more direct interpersonal discussion. A danger in these discussions is that some people would use the opportunity to vent hostility in the guise of helping others to understand themselves better. Because ego growth does not take place in an atmosphere of hostility, the leader must carefully control the group. To lead such a program successfully is not difficult; psychiatrists do so frequently. The failing in present activities is that there is no organization, no continuity, and no clear distinction between community mental hygiene and treatment. Businessmen plagued with personnel problems are largely unaware of the help a properly conceived and executed program could provide toward the solution of many knotty problems. The public schools, which may have consultants for teaching or evaluating the mentally ill children, have no organized mental hygiene program available, although in the author's experience teachers are eager to participate. Many universities shun the topic of mental hygiene in the schools, isolating their Department of Education from the benefits of closer cooperation with the departments of psychiatry, social work, and psychology. Thus teachers, one of the most important groups involved in the improvement of ego functioning, receive little training in this field.

The mental hygiene agency could also make its service available to individuals by conducting group sessions and seminars. A complication is that the people most likely to sign up would be those who have defective egos and need psychotherapy rather than a mental hygiene program. Some of these would drop out when they saw the program was not meeting their needs; others might remain and obtain some benefit. Even with a diversified group a skillful leader could keep the session productive, and this skill is now available among the psychologically trained people in any large community. If the sessions were run for a short time, they would be primarily a direct educational experience; they could, however, be extended into discussion groups.

Thus the mental hygiene agency would offer broad and inclusive services. It should have a clearly defined purpose, be easily available, and be prepared to offer a series of programs tailored to the demands and levels of all the various groups within the community who might wish to avail themselves of its service.

Implementation of the Mental Hygiene Agency

The mental hygiene agency would need a full-time director, preferably a psychiatrist experienced in working with groups, teaching, and conducting discussions. The remaining personnel would be drawn from the pool of trained people in any large community and employed on a contract basis as they were needed. In time, the agency would have available a number of specialists working with various kinds of groups. There would be no need for many full-time people; in fact, too many might stultify the agency. A large pool of interested consultants would provide the constant innovation necessary for a vital, efficient program.

Financial Support

The agency should be operated as part of the state mental hygiene program in conjunction with interested communities. In California, the state spends $121,000,000 annually to care for the mentally ill. No money is now allocated for improving the egos of those who don't function anywhere near their best, although it seems certain that as the general level of ego functioning rises, there will be fewer mentally ill. A small part of the state mental hygiene budget would be sufficient to start mental hygiene programs in California's largest cities.

Research and statistics in this field have progressed sufficiently to permit an evaluation of the success of a mental hygiene program. After ten to fifteen years, if the program worked, there should be a reduction in the number of mentally ill. We might also expect a change in the quality of mental illness—that is, fewer seriously defective patients, and a greater percentage of patients with milder ego defects. A further advantage is that more people would receive benefits from the positive side of psychiatry, a direct advantage to the average citizen who has up to now seen this portion of his taxes spent only for the mentally ill.

Facilities

Extensive facilities would not be required because the agency personnel would be sent out to interested organizations. Avoiding the rigid confines of an institution, the personnel would learn to work flexibly in the field. The group sessions and programs for interested individuals would attain greater psychological impact if existing community facilities such as schools, churches, union halls, and industrial auditoriums, were used. Using a wide variety of meeting places in the community would increase the chances of bringing mental hygiene to the people whom it might benefit.

Although this discussion of mental hygiene is brief, it is hoped it will help to open avenues now clogged by thinking only of treatment. Treatment is always important, but in an ideal community treatment would eventually become secondary to a proper program of mental hygiene. This transition has already occurred in many diseases where prevention has long since replaced extensive treatment programs. Smallpox, whooping cough, diphtheria and, hopefully, soon polio are a few of these diseases; cancer and heart disease may join the list within this century. In considering mental illness, however, the present emphasis is on treatment. Unfortunately, there is little organized clamor for a different approach through a mental hygiene program, possibly along the lines introduced here.

Conclusion

It was the purpose of this book to shed light on the problems of mental illness, to explain clearly and systematically how effective as well as defective people function, and to show what psychiatry does and should do to help solve these problems. Knowledge will help sweep away the unnecessary ignorance-caused stigma often associated with mental illness. It is the hope of the author that people will demand more and better psychiatric treatment, that public pressure will require higher standards of institutional care, that in certain cases, psychiatric treatment will supersede criminal prosecution, and that each community will initiate a mental hygiene program to begin to attack the sources of mental illness.

Index

Acceptance of treatment, 95, 99, 135, 152, 156-161, 169, 184-185
Achievement, need for, 6
Aggression, as ego function, 17-19
    relation to racial prejudice, 38
    sexual, 110-111
Alcoholism, 94-95
    and personality disorders, 68-69
    and psychosis, 127-128
Anger, and boredom, 31
    and depression, 30-31, 129, 182-183
    as ego reaction, 28-29
    harmful influences of, 130
    of mother, 48
    and poor ego functioning, 28-29
    and psychosomatic disease, 134-138
    and psychophysiologic reactions, 31-32
Anxiety, as basic ego reaction, 22-24, 27-30
    in character disorders, 66-67
    and character neurotics, 93, 98-99
    and compulsion, 41
    lack of, 23-24, 66-67, 84, 85, 93
    neurosis, 71-74, 89-92
    purpose of, 24
    and sexual confusion, 100-102, 103-104, 106, 109-110
    and symptom neurosis, 79-88; *see also* Hostility
Asthma, 138
Atmosphere, therapeutic, 152-153, 170-174, 177, 179

"Beatniks," 26
Behavior, forceful aggressive, 17-19
    normal, 1

Boredom, 31
Borrowing, ego, 54-55, 68-69

Character; *see* Personality
Character disorder, 60-68, 96, 170-175
Character neurosis, 82-100
Child, developing ego function of, 43-50
    raising, 192-199
Children, psychiatric treatment of, 160-161
    psychosis in, 117-118, 121, 128-129
    and realism, 74-75
Claustrophobia, 81-83
Cleanliness mania, 41
Clinics, for heroin addicts, 177-178
    psychiatric, 149, 152
Clinical psychologists, 146-147
Colitis, 135, 137-138
Compulsion, 41, 86-88
Conversion reaction, 83-84, 85
Cost of caring for mentally ill, 111-112, 202
Criminals, sexual, 102, 103, 108, 109-111; *see also* Delinquents
    white-collar, 97-98

Danger of psychotic patients, 110-111, 180
Dean, James, 26
Death, and anger, 131-133, 134, 136, 138, 139; *see also* Suicide
Defects, ego, in parents, 52
Defense, denial as, 37-38; *see also* Denial *and* Sublimation
    ego, 33-35
Delinquents, adult, 174-175

INDEX

Delinquents, juvenile; *see* Juvenile delinquents
Dementia praecox, 117
Denial, 37-38
Depression, and anger, 129-140
  as basic ego reaction, 22, 30-31
  defined, 30
  institutional treatment of, 182-184
  shock treatments for, 153
Destructiveness and emptiness, 63
Discipline, corporal, 198
  school, 197
Disease
  hypochondriacal, 85-86
  psychosomatic, 31-32, 134-140
Disorders, character, 60-68, 96, 170-175
Dreams, as ego defenses, 34-35
Drug addiction, 65-66, 176-178; *see also* Heroin
Drugs, and acting-in neuroses, 95-97
  psychiatric tranquilizing, 153-154
Drunkenness, 94-95

Eczema, 139
Education, mental hygiene as, 188, 200, 201
Ego, and anger, 28-29, 130
  borrowed, 54-55, 68-69
  of character neurotics, 93-94
  of child, 43-50
  defective, 51-53
  defined, 9
  development of, 42-55
  effective, 27, 50-51
  fragmented, 60-69
Ego defense, personality as, 41
  tasks of, 33-35
Ego function, affected by gaps, 61-69
  borrowed, 53-55, 68-69
  and depression, 30
  and emotions, 20-23
  improving, 10
  and phobia, 82-83
  primary, 10-12, 13
  and psychosis, 112-117, 119
Ego strengthening, psychiatrist and, 162-163, 164-169
Emotions as basic ego reactions, 22
  of child, 48-49
  of parents, 197-199
  as reward of effective ego functioning, 20-23

Emptiness, as basic ego reaction, 22, 24-27
  due to gaps in ego, 63-69
  of heroin addicts, 176
  and homosexuals, 105-106
Environment, 42-43; *see also* Atmosphere *and* Reality

Father, relationship of, with child, 49; *see also* Mother *and* Parents
Fear, as anxiety, 23
  and anxiety neurosis, 72-74, 89-92
  and character neurotics, 93
  and female homosexuals, 106
  and sex, 77
Food addict, 97
Frustration of child, 194-195, 196

Gamblers, 97
Gang, juvenile, 64
Grief and anger, 131-132
Group therapy, 174, 175-176, 181
Guilt, as anxiety, 23

Hallucinations, 112
Heredity, 42-43
Heroin, 65-66, 96; *see also* Drugs
  addicts of in institutions, 176-177
Hives, 138-139
Home, two-way relationships in, 67-68; *see also* Father, Mother *and* Parents
Homosexuality, frequency of, 78
  latent, 108
  pseudo-, 65
Homosexuals, 102-108
  female, 101-102, 106-108
  in institutions, 175
  and marriage, 105, 110
Hospitals, mental, 111, 178
  staff of, 146-149
Hostility, as basic ego reaction, 22
  and emptiness, 25-26
  expressed by effective egos, 27
Hypertension, 140
Hypochondriasis, 85-86
Hysteria, 83-85

Identity, and "brainwashing," 32-33
  of child, 49
  as ego function, 13-16
  and emptiness, 24-27
  lack of, 61, 63, 64

INDEX

Identity (cont.)
  sexual, 14-15, 51, 77-78, 101, 102, 105, 108-109
Ileitis, 138
Illness, hypochondriacal, 85-86; see also Psychosomatic disease
Insight, and ego defects, 167-168

Judgment, as reality test, 16-17
Juvenile delinquents, 59-61, 63, 64, 65, 67
  emptiness, 24
  hostility, 27
  punishment, 48
  treatment in institutions, 170-171, 172-173

Lobotomy, 154
Loss, and anger, 130-132, 133
  and depression, 183
Love, and homosexuals, 102, 104
  need for, 5
  and psychosis, 117-118

Mania, cleanliness, 41
Marriage, and acting-out neurotics, 99-100
  and homosexuals, 105, 110
Masculinity; see Homosexuals *and* Sexual Identity
Men, aggressiveness of, 18-19
  sexual identity of, 14-15
Mental hygiene, defined, 187
Mental hygiene agency, 189, 199-204
Mental illness, stigma of, 157, 204
Migraine, 139-140
Money, and children, 75
Mother, and ego-borrowing of infant, 44-47
  overprotective, 131
  relationship with child, 43-48

Narcotics Anonymous, 177; see also Drug Addiction *and* Heroin
Needs, basic, 3-6
  denial of, 37
  ego, 10-11
  psychological, 4-5
  sexual, 62, 65, 69
  social, 5-6
  and sublimation, 35-37
  transmission of, 53-55, 68-69
Neuroses, acting-in, 95-97

Neuroses (cont.)
  acting-out, 97-100
  anxiety, 71-74, 78, 89-92
  character, 92-100
  hypochondriacal, 85-86
  obsessive-compulsive, 86-88
  sexual, 100-111
  symptom, 70, 71
Neurotics, anxiety, 158
  character, 158-159
  sexual, 158-159, 175-176
  symptom, 158
Normality, defined, 1
Nurses, psychiatric, 147-148
Nymphomaniac, 109

Obsessions, 86-88
"Operators," and neurosis, 97-100
Overprotection of child, 73-76, 131

Parents, and anxiety, 72-75
  defective egos in, 52
  overprotective, 73-76, 131
  role of, in mental hygiene, 188, 192-199
Peeping Tom, 102, 110, 175
"Permissiveness," 196, 198
Personality, compulsive, 41
  defined, 39-41
Perversions, sexual, 100-111
Phobia, 86
  and anxiety, 23
  and symptom neurosis, 80-83
Pleasure as reward of effective ego functioning, 20-21
Preconscious, 32, 33
Prejudice, racial, 38
"Prison code," 173, 179
Prisoners of war, and identity, 32-33
Projection; see Denial
Psychiatric social workers, training of, 146
Psychiatric treatment, defined, 141, 162-169
Psychiatrist, and character neurotics, 99
  function of, 12, 13, 41
  relation to medical doctor, 135, 137, 154, 184-185
  training of, 145, 184
Psychiatry, and psychosomatic disease, 134, 135, 136, 137, 138, 139, 140

Psychoanalyst, training of, 145-146
Psychologists, clinical, 146-147
Psychosis, acute, 123
  age at onset, 117-118
  catatonic, 126-127
  chronic, 123
  defined, 112, 115-116
  denial and, 38
  functional, 120, 121-129
  hebephrenic, 124, 127
  organic, 119-121
  paranoid, 124-126
  and reality, 122-129
  senile, 117, 120
  simple, 127-128
  treatment of, 159-160
  undifferentiated, 128
Psychosomatic disease, 31-32, 134-140
  institutional treatment of, 184
Psychotherapy, defined, 141, 162-169
  group, 151-152
  individual, 150-151
  problems of, 155-161
Psychotic, toxic, 120-121
Punishment, corporal, 29
  of delinquents, 48

Rape, and defective ego, 62
Rationalization, and anxiety, 91-92;
  see also Denial
Realism and children, 74-75
Reality, and character neurotics, 93;
  see also Denial
  defined, 7-9
  and judgment, 16
  perception of, 23
  and psychosis, 112-116, 118-119, 122-129
  and sexual neurosis, 100
  and time concept, 16-17
Repression; see Denial
Responsibility, of child, 49, 194-195
  parental, 192-197
Restitution, psychotic, 125
Riesman, David, 25
Rorschach test, 22

Satyr, 109
Schizophrenia, 121-123
  catatonic, 124, 125, 126-127
  hebephrenic, 124, 127
  paranoid, 124, 125-126

Schizophrenia (cont.)
  simple, 124, 127-128
Self-worth, lack of, 25
Sex, need for sexual relations, 4-5;
  see also Homosexuality, Homosexuals, and Sexual identity
  and juvenile delinquents, 65
  and neurosis, 76-78, 100-111
Sexual identity, 14-15, 77-78, 101, 102, 105, 108-109
Shock, electric, 153, 182-183
Social workers, training of psychiatric, 146
Spock, Dr. Benjamin, 193
Staff, hospital, 148-149, 172-173, 179-181
Sublimation, 35-37
  mourning as, 131
Suicide, and depression, 132-133, 183
Surgery, 154
Swindlers, 97-98
Symptom neuroses, 79-88
Symptoms, psychosomatic, 31-32

Tantrums, 194, 196, 197
Technicians, psychiatric, 148
Tension, and anxiety, 23
  released by emotions, 193, 198-199
Thematic Apperception Test, 22
Therapeutic atmosphere; see Atmosphere
Thieves, 97
Time, concept of, 16-17
Tobacco addiction, 96-97
Transition homes, 175, 181-182
Treatment, acceptance of, 95, 99, 135, 152, 156-161, 169, 184-185
  in institutions, 169-185
  obstacles to, 156-157
  physical-chemical, 153-154
  psychological, 150-153

Ulcer, stomach, 136, 137-138
"Unconscious"; see Preconscious
Urticaria, 138-139

Values, as identity factor, 15

Women, aggressiveness of, 18-19
  and homosexuality, 106-108
  sexual identity of, 14-15
Work, depressed patients and, 183-184